CRACKING THE FAT CODE

Raimond Strazdins
CHPT, CWBP

The Content, including without limitation information relating to medical and health conditions, products and treatments, is often provided in summary or aggregate form. It is not intended as a substitute for advice, diagnosis or treatment from your Healthcare Professional.

Copyright © 2024 - CRACKING THE FAT CODE
All Rights Reserved

TABLE OF CONTENTS

ACKNOWLEDGEMENTS i
INTRODUCTION V

Code 1 The Natural Central Intelligence Systems 17
Code 2 The Maestro 27
Code 3 Patience Is A Virtue 33
Code 4 Be like a Fox - Be Resourceful 39
Code 5 Will the Circle Be Unbroken? 43
Code 6 Being Excellent 47
Code 7 Skip a workout Don't skip a meal! 51
Code 8 Fuel the engine - Whey cool! 55
Code 9 Water We Doing! 61
Code 10 Get the plunger 69
Code 11 TAPIN to your Temple 75
Code 12 Temple of doom 83
Code 13 You have the POWER 87
Code 14 Lucky #7 91
Code 15 The YEAST Beast 97
Code 16 El Fuego 101
Code 17 Creep show 105
Code 18 Farmers feed Cities - Hero or Villain? 109

Code 19 Acid trip 117
Code 20 You are a Sponge BOB square pants..................121
Code 21 The Key Masters 127
Code 22 Beige FAT is where its at 131
Code 23 The Sponge and the chimney sweep 137
Code 24 Beam me up scotty! 141
Code 25 Dive deep 151
Code 26 Order in the court 157
Code 27 Conquer nature 161
Code 28 Let the sun shine in 167
Code 29 Flow like water 171
Code 30 Gut check 175
Code 31 Wonder Cells Activate (supplements)............... 179
Code 32 Less is more 189
Code 33 To clean or not to clean 193
Code 34 Aerial Reconnaissance 197
Code 35 The lawn boy 201
Code 36 Operation Mineweeper 205
References 210

Acknowledgements

I owe a debt of gratitude for many people who have helped me,
guided me, taught me and made me who I am today, I thank you all.

My MOM a very hardheaded woman and needed to be due to her
ailments, taught me to never give up! We grew so much closer and
understood each other as we both aged, we really did appreciate each
other and enjoyed our time together. She died too early at age 66
with full blown diabetes a writer as well but never published, her book
almost got to the world.
I have her manuscripts; her book will get out to the world I will make
sure of that. Her death is a mystery of sorts just the way she wanted
it as she was an avid reader of Agatha Christie novels,
love you MOM, I see you slyly smiling from the heavens.

My FATHER many called him "Coach" one of the best examples of
what being a man is. He never discouraged always allowed whether I
failed or not always teaching, encouraging, always sharing, such
unconditional LOVE.
My DAD was so debonair wearing a suit so proper and cordial always
with a smile rarely a frown. Growing up on a small farm with ten
siblings it was tough. He was however the Diamond, the shining light
amongst all of the children he being the third youngest.
He shined as a small child, in athletics to playing the trumpet in a band.
 As an adult being a VP of large corporations, to owning his own
business firm consulting for large corporations.
My father showed persistence, dedication and doing it all with such
class, thank you dad.
I miss you here on the earthly plane, DAD I know you're
shining down on me sounding your trumpet from above when I most
need it.
My FATHER - my biggest HERO.

My friends who have helped me through tough times you know who
 you are, I love you all.
A special thanks to Royal for fixing my computer,
(retrieving all of my writings),this book would have never
happened if it wasn't for him. Note to all back up your work, and then
double back up your work!
So many mentors in the Wellness industry:
Deane Parkes an icon in the wellness industry and has seen it all.
 Always there to lend a hand or an ear such a leader and able to find
solutions and always finding the time, thank you.
Brad king I appreciate your friendship from afar all the books that
 you have written and all of the products that you have
formulated for companies. Such a wealth of knowledge always
 there to answer my questions if needed, thank you Brad.
Michael Crawley, you showed me the way to get this book
 finished. Thankyou for inviting me to your mentor's group this just
solidified my knowing that I had IT. And the Knowing to Just
 DO IT and finish all my books to share with the world.

So many spiritual and self awareness mentors through the years
 from Wayne Dyer, Tony Robbins, Bob Proctor, following the
philosophies of Bruce Lipton, Bruce Lee, Dale Carnegie, ·
Wallace Waddles, and Napoleon Hill to name a few.

As I went through these mentors one became very clear to me
to whom I aspire to be like as a writer.
 That writer is/was Michael Crichton he became my favorite writer.
 Michael coming from a medical background and dripping nonfiction
into his fiction novels was just brilliant.
 I love that he made you think and question things, as we all should.
 In doing so he made a lot of enemies, he pissed off a lot of people,
ruffled a lot of feathers including big corporations around the world.

If you want to talk conspiracy, I think that's why he's no
longer with us, hey that may just be in another book I write
we will see. I will aspire to be the type of fiction writer you were.
Thank you Michael Crichton I am grateful for your workings,
insights and provocations.

To my Kimberly thank you, thank you, thankyou.
The last 20 years so many ups and downs so many rocky roads and
smooth journeys so many stories so much fun!
 We have 20 years of stories; we really do it's amazing the things
we've done! So many "Lucy moments" So much more than "Just
 Another Kangaroo in Texas."
 You are my twin flame; you are such an inspiration you have helped
 so many people, your love for animals and nature, phenomenal and
so beautiful.
You mean more to me than you know, my twin flame I
thank you for everything I will always love you, and our journey
continues!
     Lastly and the most important I thank YHWH (Yahwey) – God!
The universe is so divine we get lost sometimes but as Wayne Dyer
 used to say "Let go and let God". It took me over 3 decades to
finally put the pen to paper, to print!
I thought I lost it, meaning the ability to write again I mean really
 write creatively. Although this is somewhat creative writing it is
 by far not my most creative writing.
Those books, those stories will be coming out soon.
 Those decades past just meant it just wasn't time; Only Yahwey
knows but it sure is time NOW!
 I thank God every morning and I thank God every night for my
abilities to do what I love and the freedom to do so, I am so grateful
and thankful.
*"Stop, waiting for a miracle drug or a miracle pill, help yourself
 by changing your lifestyle, you are the Miracle"*
                                        Raimond Strazdins

Introduction

Achieve Body Harmony For Your Best Weight
Was to be my book title when I started writing it , kinda does fit
but, CRACKING THE FAT CODE just made more sense to me.

This wasn't my first plan or my thought of a first book but as we
know things just happen and the universe provides end the end this
really ended up making sense to be my first non- fiction book.

We always tend to question ourselves and for me at first thought,
why would anyone want to read another weight LOSS book
there's a ton of fat loss/weight loss books diet books etc etc and
why another one.
True this is another one, alas another one with a different
perspective and this one showing the bigger picture!
I think with my 30 plus years as a Holistic Personal Trainer and
8 years as a Cell Well-Being Practitioner that time has groomed
me to SEE the bigger picture.
A different way of getting you from point A to point B really the
right way if you put all the pieces together.
For many this will resonate with them for others just another book.
I am however grateful and glad that I can help those that follow and
utilize all of the CODES.

A few QUESTIONS to ask yourself:
The first Question should be, WHY – What is your Why?

Why do you want to proceed on this journey? Put it Down on paper
-YOUR WHY IS IMPORTANT!
Second Question What are the benefits if you get to your target
Weight?

THE BENEFITS, write it DOWN.
"if you fail to plan, you plan to fail"

We were all given 24 hours a day develop a Can Do attitude. As Wayne Dyer said "Excuses Be Gone".
(great book by the way).

Make A plan of attack, be a Wellness Warrior – And follow it:
Grab a notebook, binder, mobile App. whatever – and put "Pen to Paper"!
As I have learned over the years you have to put it down on paper. This MAKES IT REAL
It's putting action into the idea; it is putting the "I want to", into I WILL – Your superhero WILLPOWER!

TFA -Everything starts with THOUGHT, we put FEELING behind it and then we must take ACTION for the manifesting to transpire. As you embark on your new journey and if you fall off the plan. SO, WHAT!!!! Get back on that WELLNESS TRAIN Get Going AGAIN – Do NOT STOP.
Make a plan - follow the plan make it a habit!
JUST KEEP GOING. I started writing stories in 1987 –that's right! WTF(Where'd Time Fly)
37 years AGO…This is my next JOURNEY it only took 37 YEARS
I have over 40 books started, and as I was writing this book more came to mind, no joke and they WILL get Out to the WORLD.
DONOT ever say NEVER sure life gets in the way, just Don't STOP! This is my 1st of many! They say the first of anything is the hardest, and I am learning as a published writer NOW as I go.
This may be my messy start as a published writer. So be it, you know the great Nike saying, "JUST DO IT".

It doesn't matter here I am… doing what I always wanted to DO and
truly believe what I am supposed to Do!
 I just finally told myself that I WILL.

That was and is the difference…The WILL not the I Want!
(a lot of little stories in there for sure)
At the end of the day - it is ALL YOU!
Be a Jedi - A Jedi Wellness Warrior – lets USE some Jedi MIND tricks
for real. Use the FORCE (Your subconscious Mind).

You can scratch the surface of that subconscious Mind
if you do positive affirmations DAILY!
Ya ya ya, blah blah blah you may have heard this before.
Let me ask you this? Has it hindered you, has it harmed you?
A big NO it hasn't.
Affirming thoughts most likely helped you and you didn't even
 know it. There are some days we need to do these affirmations
 every hour and sometimes more than that but in any event put them
into your daily schedule, put them on sticky notes on your fridge
mirrors, cupboards or wherever you may see them daily.

This can ONLY help as you journey to your optimal health
Wellness and YOUR perfect BODY!
 Humans go through 60,000 thoughts a day and on average 70%
 of those are negative. That's right negative, it seems you can do nine
things good and one thing bad. What do people generally remember?
You got it the BAD or negative. A shame really most of the time
people standing around chatting with peers, the subject always tends to
gravitate toward the negative aspects of the subject.
 Then the next day we go through the same 80% or more thoughts.
You are doomed from the start IF you continue to stay tapped into
that subconscious negative mind set.
We must keep striving for a positive frame of Mind.

Yes this is a constant battle we all must work on, but it is a MUST.
Our computer mind, this is important to note and needs to sink in.
Our conscious mind is like a 60-bit processor the subconscious
mind is like a 40-million-bit processor.
So, as you can tell the power is in the subconscious mind our own
auto pilot, the GPS, the habitual mind and our belief systems which
trip us up everyday if we let it.
Heard of PSYCH-K? This is a non-invasive process of
change. It's a simple yet powerful way of changing subconscious
beliefs that are self sabotaging and self limiting.

Using various tools for change coming from contemporary
neuroscience research it's an amazing approach to facilitate
change at the subconscious level.
I'm very grateful I was able to do my beginners my advanced
and my master's in 2020 with great teachers from
the PSYCH-K Centre INTERNATIONAL.
Thankyou teachers!
If you want to or need to go deeper to help facilitate those changes tha
you can't seem to break called habits or your BS (belief sytsems)
find yourself a facilitator or, take the basic course it is amazing
and will change your compass into the right direction and life
guaranteed.
https://psych-k.com/

"IF YOU CHANGE THE WAY YOU LOOK AT
THINGS, THE THINGS YOU LOOK AT CHANGE"
– WAYNE DYER

love this saying and its - so TRUE!
Make your Want to - I WILL
This is your ENERGY your WILLPOWER .Your FORCE!

x

Every chapter (in this book I call chapters, CODES) I put some
affirming positive thoughts that have been around for a long time.
Some that have helped me, helped many before me and helped
many get to their goals, whether a champion chess player a pro
athlete or a billionaire.
The mind game is a big piece of the CODE.
In sports they say 80% is mental 20% physical. The 80/20 rule
 (the Pareto principle)
  When you do these affirmations you want to put action into it, this
anchors them flowing into the subconscious mind more easily.
 I like to call them declarations, your Declaration of Independence!
 As you do these declarations put your hand on your heart
 (connecting body mind and soul) take a deep breath and exhale
and say them with meaning.
 I have done affirmations and declarations for years and they
really do work. They tend to keep you in a positive space and much
 needed when you feel down, they lift you up, focused and centered
they really do. Just closing your eyes or focusing on an object and
saying a few things in a positive way can get you out of that
downward negative energy and turning our day into a brighter one.

 Wayne Dyer Louise Hay, Bob Proctor, Harv Eker, Tony Robbins
 and many others all talk about these affirmations/declarations and
 the importance of them.
 I do my affirmations/declarations every day. They have helped me
through some dark times, providing me with a great start to the day.
Now as I get up in the wee hours of the morning when my feet hit
the floor the first words out of my mouth are "how may I serve"
 It's a great way to start the Day! I picked this beautiful idea and
mantra up from one of my mentor's Dr. Wayne Dyer.

 There was no way I could write a book without having these
declarations amongst the pages as I provide solutions
throughout.

Cracking the CODE: As I wrote cracking the FAT CODE I wanted the book to be as short and concise as much as possible.
 Just cracking each chapter in which I will call CODES: giving a glimpse of what is possible with solutions and insights.
I hope you find some gold nuggets in Cracking the FAT code!
 The first declaration I will write is..
oh wait. wait… put down the device/book and let's put some action to this shall we. Take a deep breathe in, hold for 5 seconds and release let it out.
Put your hand on your heart and say:
"my inner world creates my outer world".
 You may think or feel this a bit goofy?
So WHAT lets have some FUN here and see where it leads shall WE…
Awesome and so it begins, let's dive in , may the force be with you!

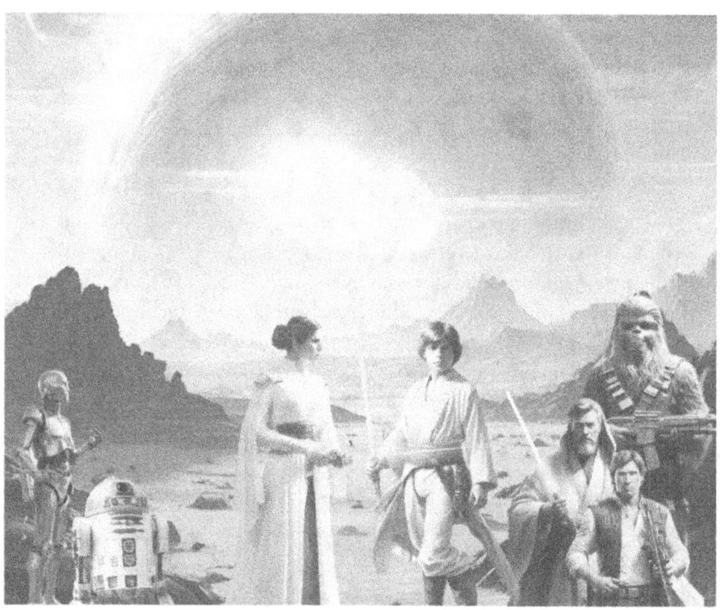

THE BIG PICTURE

The Human Body Machine:

50 trillion Cells within these are 30 billion Fat Cells

Fun fact - Did You Know That 99.9% of All Humans DNA Is the Same?

Did you know that They cracked the human genome code?

The human Genome project had a soft start in 1987 but formally began in October 1990 and completed in 2003. When it ended it was a bit of a WTG moment.

It ended with many more questions than they started with. Their assumptions from many studies, hours, days, months, years of lab testing etc. they figured and assumed on about 100,000 genes to 150,000 genes when the project ended.

The great WTG -Where's The Genes...moment!

What they ended up finding was around 25,000 genes a far cry from 100,000 plus genes they had expected.

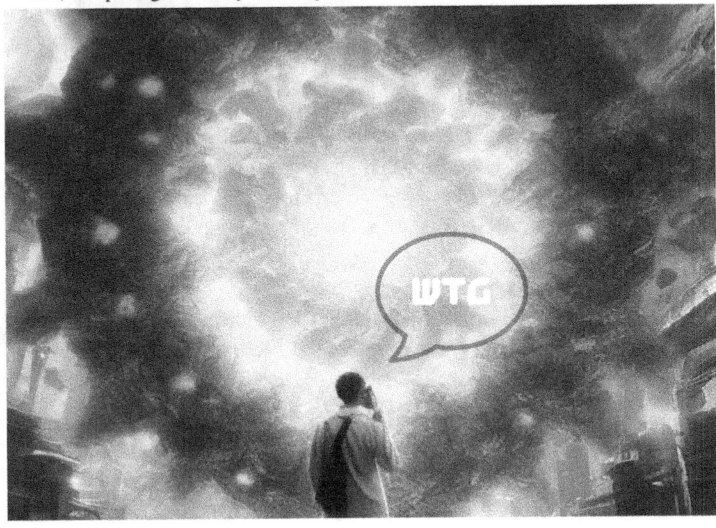

To top it off there where just 1,000 more genes then a little WORM!

The Caenorhabditis elegans a miniature worm a very small organism barely visible with your eye with around 1200 cells to the human 50 trillion cells? Huh? So, where oh where are all the other cells?
The conventional medicine advocates didn't know and still don't know and are still searching.

One of my favorite Mentors Dr. Bruce Lipton knows and knew way before the project started in 1987 and he talks about it to this day!

Its based on EPIGENETICS – for further deeper explanation A Few books to dive into are "The Wisdom Of Your Cells" and "The Biology of Belief" by Dr. Bruce Lipton
It explains the whole Medical conundrum including the Genome project.

In interviews the Medical establishment acknowledges but doesn't pursue or shall I say lead the public to see it this way .
The new understanding is that environmental signals to regulatory protein then to DNA then to RNA and then to protein.
Why is it relevant? DNA is not at the top of that information scheme the **Environment** is.

Unfortunately, Allopathic (conventional) medicine still says we control the genes and are still under the spell of...
"Lets dominate nature".

Code: One

NCIS – Natural Central Intelligence Systems

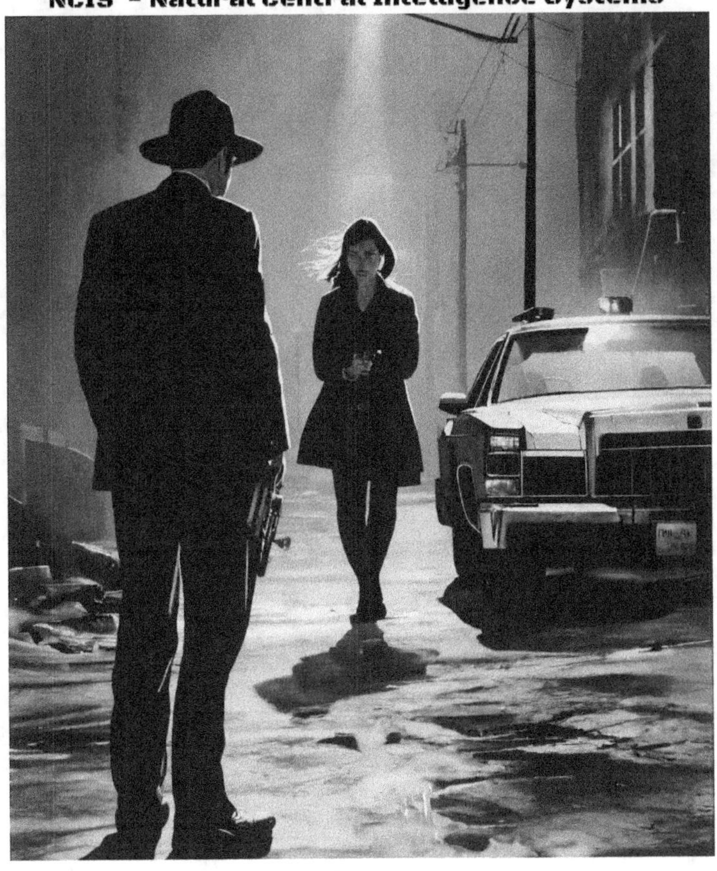

Natural Intelligence Systems

CRACKING THE FAT CODE

Our Focus: Lets Just Get one thing very CLEAR, "Focus Daniel Son", my Mr Miyagi voice. From the Karate Kid movies of the 1980's. This is important and needs to get you thinking differently. I must report what many Don't, or Won't and generally fail to realize, we do not ever lose FAT cells, that's right Ever!
You are born with approximately 30 billion cells, and you will die with the same 30 billion cells.
The only way you lose them is by getting them sucked out your body via liposuction. To me this is a very bad idea since you were created with everything you need for an abundant healthy Life.
Yep spoiler alert, onward we have these 30 billion FAT cells for life and will stay with us until we expire.
All the FAT loss gurus and supplement companies out in the world are kinda lying to you if they don't really tell you what's going on and giving you the full cellular NCIS picture.
Its entirely how the FAT cells are utilized and function throughout your life. We want them to perform and operate as they should and at a nominal size , yes, size matters.
A FAT cell can expand 1000 times its size lets not do that shall we lets normalize the FAT cells and have them work efficiently
the way they were designed.

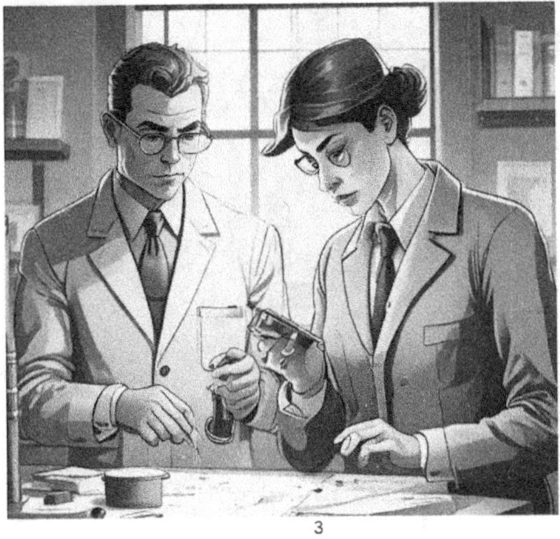

Natural Central Intelligence Systems

CRACKING THE FAT CODE

Time to investigate:
NCIS – Natural Central Intelligence Systems
All SYSTEMS Go
The Human body has an ENERGY SYSTEM actually 3 systems.
 Many business mentors will tell you to build your business you must
have systems in place to scale up your businesses, this also applies to
the human body and how efficiently it runs!
Systems must be in place and work efficiently if you want to succeed.
 Some explanation on these before we go through the
 waist land of :WHY NOTS of FAT LOSS and WEIGHT LOSS.

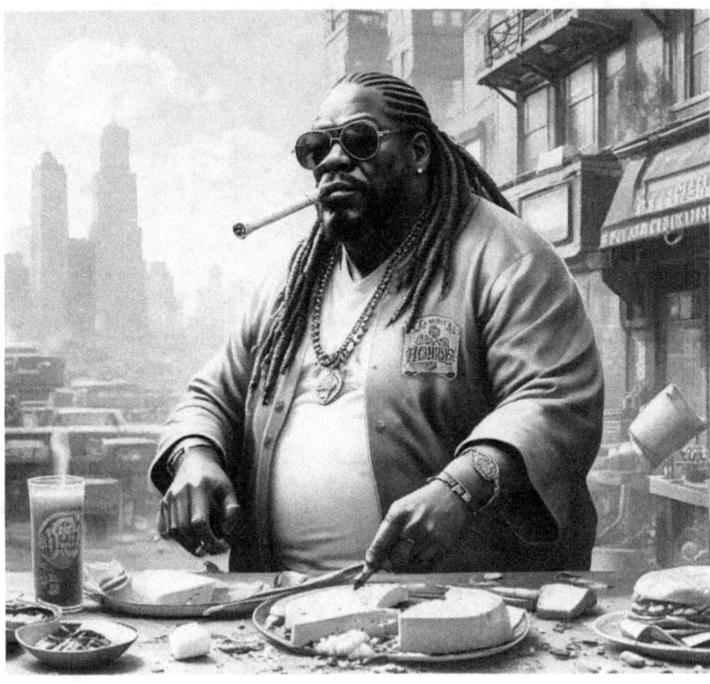

Natural Central Intelligence Systems

SYSTEM 1

Phosphagen System (ATP-CP) - this system provides immediate energy also known as ATP (Adenosine triphosphate) primarily for short-term, high-intensity activities, like sprinting and is active at the start point of any exercise.

I was introduced to ATP in the 1990's and the dawn of Creatine supplements!

I became a sales Rep for a nutraceutical company out of Toronto, Canada and probably sold more creatine than anyone in Southwestern Ontario for a spell. I was passionate about it knew it worked and loved the science behind it.

Therefore, I had no issue with endorsing the product to customers and clients and I still due to this day there are no issues or side effects to note nothing but positive feedback.

Creatine helps you rev up and restore your ATP and to this day I implement Creatine in my personalized natural energy drink daily.

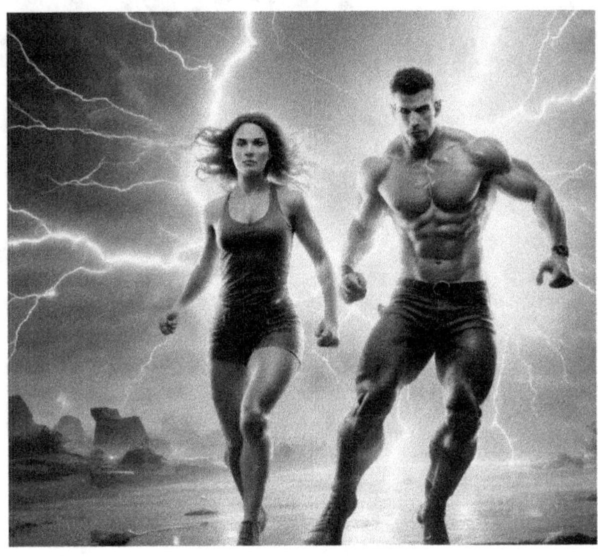

People constantly hear me talking about Creatine and its importance for all. This is one supplement that many just don't know or think about and should, the benefits are impeccable.

Both men and woman can utilize this amazing supplement.

Creatine is a go for ages 12 and up, seniors are seeing great benefits from this as well!

Many studies show the multiple benefits!

In a 2011 study they showed positive effects for the elderly and their cognitive function.

Its not just for bodybuilders and athletes as many seem to think.

No it won't get you bloated big and bulky or make you look like Arnold, but it will help you in many ways.

– always go for quality do not go cheap!

Checkout recommendations in the supplement Code 31.

SYSTEM 2

- The Glycolytic System - central metabolic pathway that is used by all cells for the oxidation of glucose to generate energy in the form of ATP it is the go between for other metabolic pathways.

This is the dominate system for most sports like : Hockey, football, sprinting, cycling, tennis and mixed martial arts to name a few.

Since glucose is the most important energy source for us it makes this system crucial and more importantly it is the only fuel for red blood cells.

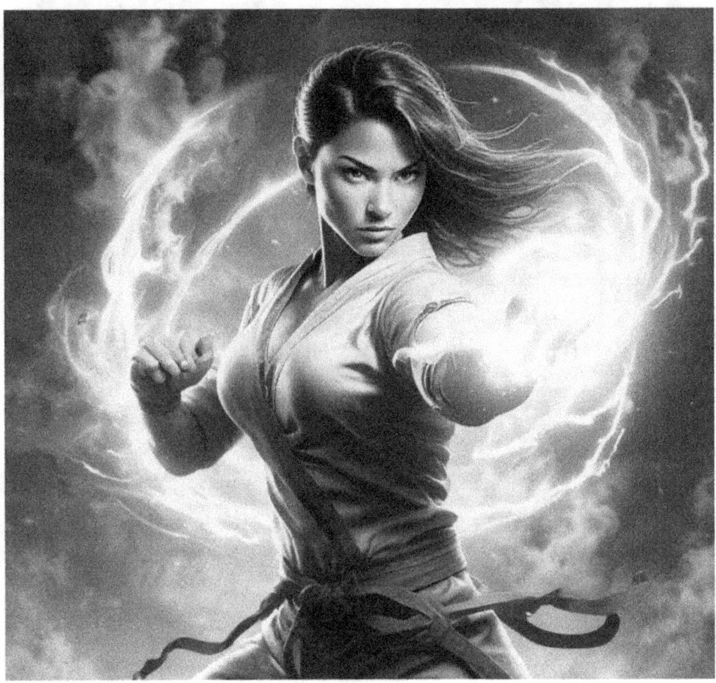

SYSTEM 3

- The Oxidative System - During low-intensity activities, uses primarily carbohydrates and fats as the foundation. Following the onset of activity, as the intensity of exercise increases, there is a shift in the key preference from fats to carbohydrates.
This is quite valuable to note and is why tons of sport science shows how the HIIT (High intensity interval training) works so well.
 This method of workouts using resistance exercises with aerobic exercises burn the most calories and use all of the energy systems.

Over many years I have trained a lot of clients utilizing cardio Kickboxing with compound 2-minute (my version of HIIT) resistance exercises with profound results.
Something to consider as you start your exercise program.
 Your going to start one right?

OK - Declaration Time!

Declaration: Put your Hand on your Heart and say:

" I am Happy, Healthy, Strong FULL of LOVE and LIGHT!"

CODE: TWO

The MAESTRO

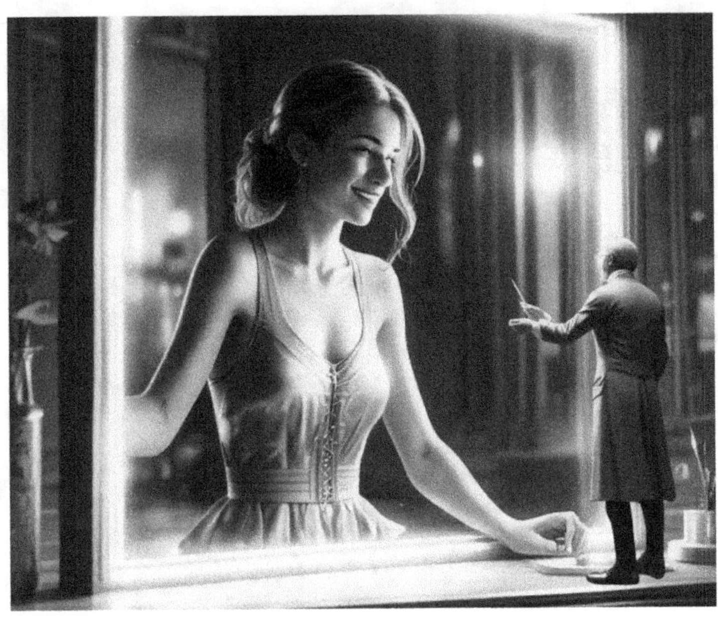

The Maestro

CRACKING THE FAT CODE

Ok maestro - Body Composition

It's all about Body Composition
  Remember the human body can be a FAT burning machine, but it all depends on the calories that are being introduced into the body and the ones being burned off daily from the body.

Regular exercise, avoiding toxins and processed food can and will help our bodies engage in the fat burning process.

Measurements Please

- Over the years of training clients, I always used the body impedance machine instead of the scale.
Technically called - Bioelectrical impedance analysis (BIA)
Showing body composition, in particular body fat, muscle mass and water.
It does so by inducing a weak electric current which flows through the body and the voltage is measured.
 The Product I used was The professional unit from Tanita, one of the highest quality units out in the market back in the 1990's.
 They now have quite a large selection to choose from these days.

The Maestro

For the love of all that's good and decent don't Do it.
Don't get on the scale in the morning everyday just don't do it.

Instead of looking at a scale, which really doesn't give you much
indication of what is going on inside the body, go with the better
indicators.
The old school type scale gives you a weight of whatever, the scale
doesn't give you much of an indicator and doesn't tell you what is
actually working within the body.

I chose and still choose the BIM (body impedance machine).
 As a matter of fact back in the day I told my clients to not look at
their scale to put it away and better yet throw the damn thing out!

I felt and I still feel the scale does more harm than good unless your
weighing GOLD .

The Maestro

If you're looking at the scale daily and you're going up and down like a yoyo you just see yourself adding another pound everyday well it becomes nothing but a negative stress.

The negative statements you say to yourself and yelling at the scale just puts stress upon yourself its detrimental and Cortisol goes up! Really it becomes a really bad habit so "Say No" to a Scale.

It's the body composition that matters anyway!

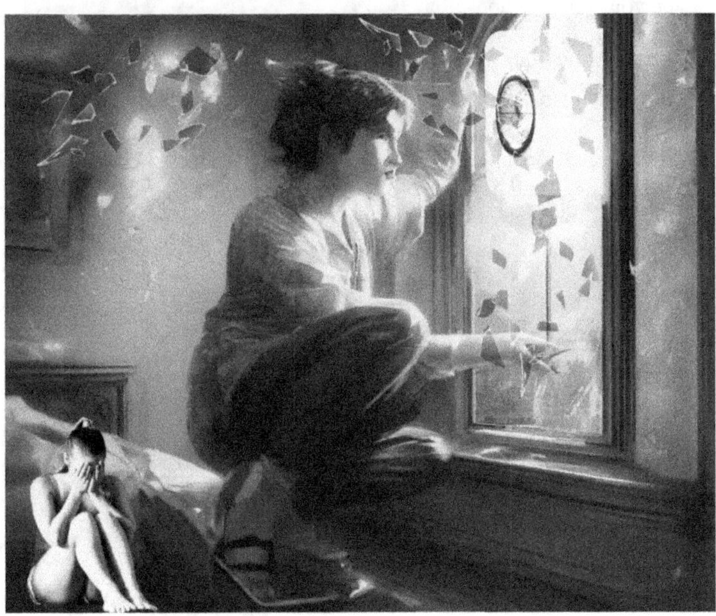

CRACKING THE FAT CODE

Many trainers use the skin calipers over the body impedance machine because of the expense and lugging around the machine. The calipers are a good measuring tool, a good tool if done correctly. You can buy some and do it yourself.

With the calipers we must get the same spot each time the trainer should do the measurements three or four times then take the mean average of all the results, its a little more time consuming but is the only accurate way to do it.

This to me is why the body impedance machine is the easier way to go it tells us how much fat muscle and how much water our body has on a readout with all the calculations done, math not my favorite subject anyway.

The newer TECH on the market makes it way easier to get a handle on your body composition.

There are units that are quite reasonable out in the market now not like my old $3500.00 TANITA in the 1990s most now have Apps you can use on your phone and log your progress to your desired Body weight.

This should be done only once a week or every other week. It's how your jeans fit and how you look in the mirror when you're naked that tells you that you're on the right path or not.

Again the scale doesn't matter it's your body composition and how you feel in your own skin.

Declaration: Put your Hand on your Heart and say:

"I am beautiful, body, mind and spirit"

CODE: THREE

PATIENCE IS A VIRTUE

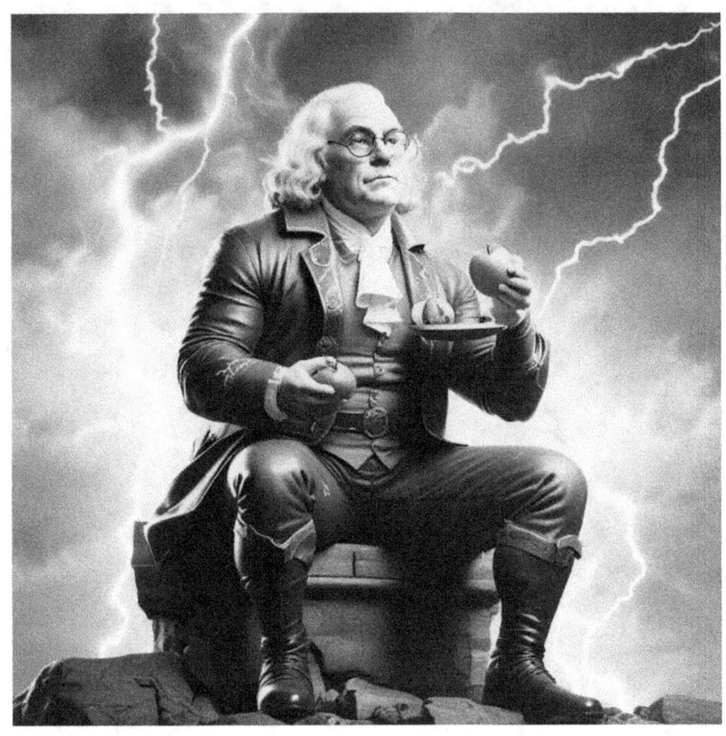

Patience Is A Virtue

VIRTUE – PATIENCE IS A VIRTUE

– Although Ben didn't include "Patience" in his 13 Virtues, I believe it is just as important, I love the timeless LIFE VIRTUES of the great Ben Franklin they do bode well on this journey!

1.**TEMPERANCE**: Eat not to dullness; drink not to elevation.

2. **SILENCE**: Speak not but what may benefit others or yourself; avoid trifling conversation.

3. **ORDER**: Let all your things have their places; let each part of your business have its time.

4. **RESOLUTION**: Resolve to perform what you ought; perform without fail what you resolve.

5. **FRUGALITY**: Make no expense but to do good to others or yourself, i.e., waste nothing.

6. **INDUSTRY**: Lose no time; be always employed in something useful; cut off all unnecessary actions.

7. **SINCERITY**: Use no hurtful deceit; think innocently and justly, and, if you speak, speak accordingly.

8. **JUSTICE**: Wrong no one by doing injuries or omitting the benefits that are your duty.

9. **MODERATION**: Avoid extremes; forbear resenting injuries so much as you think they deserve.

10. **CLEANLINESS**: Tolerate no uncleanliness in body, clothes, or habitation.

11. **TRANQUILLITY**: Be not disturbed at trifles, or at accidents common or unavoidable.

12. **CHASTITY**: Rarely use venery(act, or practice) but for health or offspring, never to dullness, weakness, or the injury of your own or another's peace or reputation.

13. **HUMILITY**: Imitate Jesus and Socrates.

- Great Virtues to live by -

Patience Is A Virtue

Doing too much all at once and expecting things to change in a day,
the human body is an amazing machine but not that good…
slow and steady. Have patience, slow and controlled.

 A BIG NO! You can't get to your preferred state of Body Mind and
Soul from ordering on Amazon and having It delivered at your
doorstep the next day!
 Society has been trying to push us into, "I need it NOW!" mentality
don't acquiesce to this hold firm to the plan, your plan.

Rome wasn't built in a day, and you didn't get where you are in a
day either. Too many times people jump on the weight loss/fat
loss/keto/carnivore etc. band wagons and go at it like sprinter with
an all or nothing NOW or nothing attitude!
We have all heard the term "baby steps" it is a journey, enjoy it!
Take the baby steps, then you can walk, then you can run.
 This is so important! Slow and Steady...

This is a marathon not a Sprint as is life. Its a way of life we all have
24 hours in a day so there is no excuse that WE don't have enough
time. WE just need to take the time.

 It's really about taking the time for YOU and to form strategies to
help YOU attain your Goal!
Pick the program that fits your style and schedule.

and……… GO FOR IT!

Patience did I say this already…..give the plan and or program a chance.
It takes 30 days to change a habit, the next 30 to really work the new habitual way of thinking and being.
 Finally, the next 30 days after that to really see how the new way the habit feels and benefits the new you!!!

   Give yourself 90 days, thats a quarter of a year and you will be pleasantly surprised of the changes that occur once you get the ball rolling.
You didn't get to where you're at in 90 days Right?

Give yourself a break on this you are HERE and NOW.
 ..oh ya and patience is a VIRTUE!

Declaration: Put your Hand on your Heart and say:

"I Now have all the Time I need."

Patience Is A Virtue

CODE: FOUR

Be like a Fox – Be Resourceful

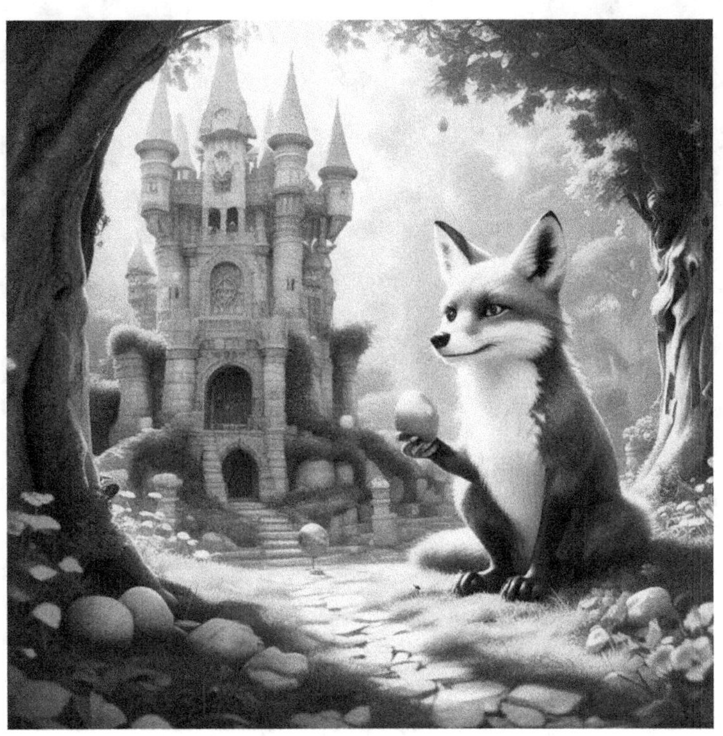

Be like a Fox - Be Resourceful

CRACKING THE FAT CODE

Be like a Fox - Be Resourceful

The Red Fox is regarded as one of the most resourceful
mammals on the planet, be like a Red Fox.
Find a resource, this book is a resource but add resources
to your journey – whether a coach, trainer, online or
other.
Most professionals have Mentors and coaches, all the
PRO sports teams have trainers and coaches. We All need
these support systems to succeed and level UP.

They need to resonate with you, and sometimes you
outgrow a mentor or coach as YOU grow. Nothing wrong
with this we need stay slightly uncomfortable, if we get
too comfortable, we become complacent.
 Don't let that happen we need to be ever growing and this
helps us to, as I tell me clients "Thrive and Optimize."
 Move to the next coach/mentor, the upside is they may
have a totally different perspective. This will enhance your
growth to find Body/Mind Harmony to get to your best
weight and best life!
To help you on your Wellness journey I have inserted the
self-confidence and worthy formula. We all need to
remind our self daily of our self-confidence and
worthiness and what our **goals truly are**. I belong to a few
mentors' groups and find them uplifting and quite helpful.
This is another resource for yourself that will assist you to
solidify your chief aim.
    Declaration: Put your Hand on your Heart and say:

    "We can achieve ANYTHING together."

Be like a Fox - Be Resourceful

1.I DEMAND of myself persistent, continuous ACTION towards its attainment, and I NOW promise to render such ACTION.

2.I realize the dominating thoughts of my mind will eventually reproduce themselves into physical REALITY. I WILL concentrate on my thoughts for 10 minutes or more daily.
UNTO the task of thinking of the person I intend to become, hereby creating in my MIND a clear and mental picture of the OPTIMAL Person I am to become.

3. I know through the principle of autosuggestion, my desire that I hold persistently in my mind will eventually seek expression through some practical means of attaining the goal/object. Therefore, I WILL devote 10 minutes daily to demanding of myself the development of SELF -CONFIDENCE and WORTHINESS.

4. I have clearly written down my description of MY DEFINITE Chief AIM of my HEALTH
and WELLESS GOAL. I WILL never stop trying, until I developed sufficient self-confidence and worthiness for its attainment.
I WILL sign my name to this formula, commit it to memory, and repeat it once a day, with full FAITH that it will gradually influence my THOUGHTS and ACTIONS so that I WILL become: Happy, healthy, strong, worthy, confident and Successful.

__________________________________ DATE

PRINT NAME

____

SIGNATURE

Chief AIM of my HEALTH and WELLESS GOAL.

CODE: FIVE

" Will the Circle Be Unbroken? "

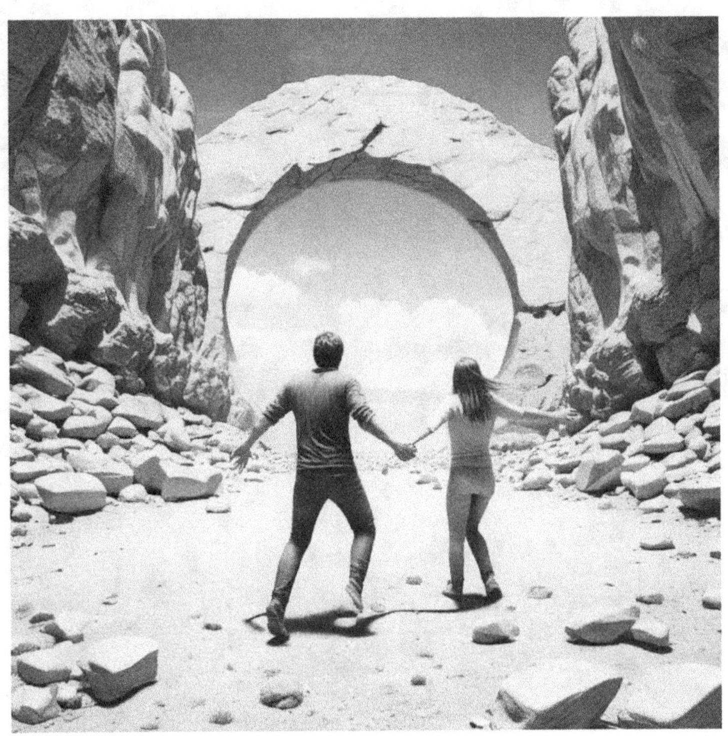

Will the Circle Be Unbroken

CRACKING THE FAT CODE

WILL THE CIRCLE BE UNBROKEN?

" Will the Circle Be Unbroken? "
 written in 1907 by Ada R. Habershon

Well - Sometimes your circle MUST be Broken for you to GROW!
Your friends circle environment (integral part of epigenetics).
All the big thinkers and high level professionals affirm that the people you hang around will dictate the person that YOU ARE and become.
 Hanging around a bunch of whiners everything is wrong, negative type people you soon become them.
Pick your friends wisely sometimes you have to break that circle and find NEW friends, those that are in the same vibrational path you're in to help you get to your goal.
Whether you are trying to get to your perfect weight, financial goal or other look around you, who are you spending your time with? Are they supportive for your wellbeing and your GOALS?
 If these so-called supporters are sitting around eating cake, bitchin, drinking, getting high, and chain smoking is this the environment for a healthy and vibrant lifestyle?
 Is it helping you achieve your goals?
A big FAT - pun intended **NO**, this does not mean you unfriend them but limit your time with them and
 follow those that inspire you to be **the Best YOU**.
  Declaration: Put your Hand on your Heart and say:

" I attract people to me who are dedicated to high integrity and LOVE"

Will the Circle Be Unbroken

CODE: SIX

Being Excellent!

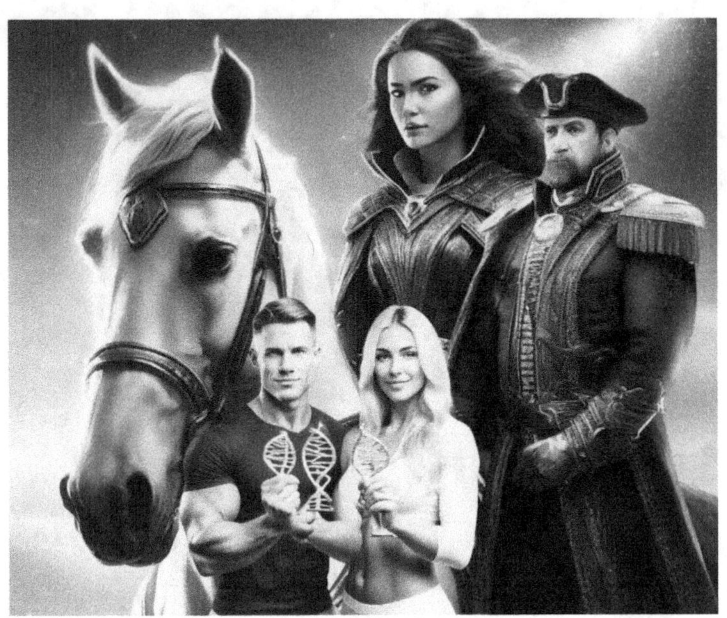

Being Excellent

CRACKING THE FAT CODE

Being Excellent

Choosing a quality and I mean quality program for your best weight and body harmony.
Not weight loss or fat loss, these are of a negative mindset and that is why there a 95% failure rate!!!

This has not changed in 50 plus years the failure rate is still 95%
I kinda think we gotta change the paradigm – right? RIGHT!

The body doesn't want to lose anything well most things.
The body wants to gain harmony and homeostasis this being the correct Paradigm.

Homeostasis: The state of steady internal, physical, chemical, and social conditions maintained by living systems.
Three great examples of this is Blood pressure regulation, Blood sugar regulation, and Body temperature (one of the reasons our body holds onto certain types of FAT).

There are many facets to **"doing things in a certain way"** and doing things at an easy pace.
 The turtle and the hare (Achilles and the tortoise) paradox comes to mind.
Time to excel, leave behind the old ways, they didn't work (not for very long)
DO THINGS IN A CERTAIN WAY
New paradigm, time to be Excellent!

Declaration: Put your Hand on your Heart and say:

"everyday in everyway I achieve excellence and harmony"

Being Excellent

CODE: SEVEN

Skip a workout Don't skip a meal!

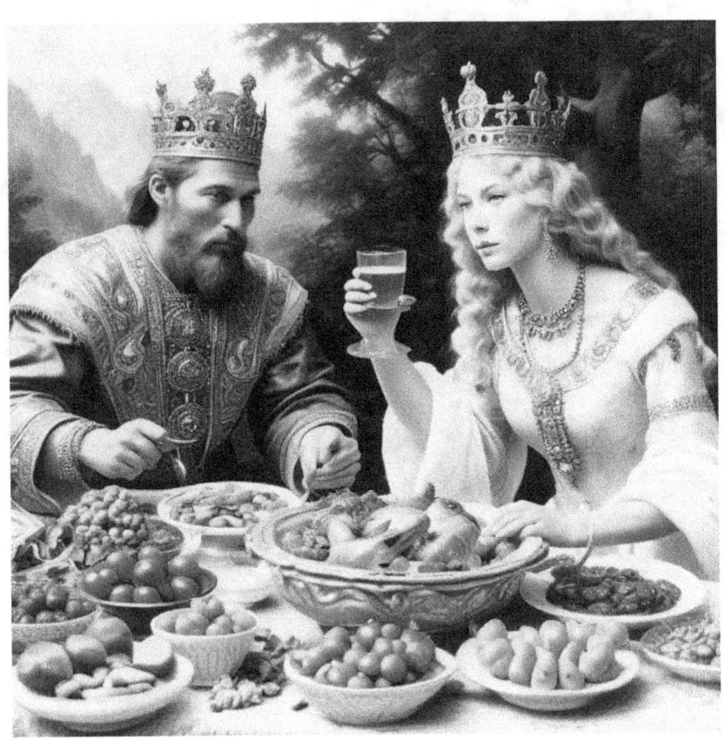

Skip a workout Don't skip a meal

CRACKING THE FAT CODE

Skip a workout Don't skip a meal!

Skipping meals: a BIG No-No!
I was taught years ago its better to skip your workout than to miss a
meal. We want to make sure that the protein and other nutrient
intake is adequate to sustain you for the day.

Unless you are doing intermittent fasting – which works well for
some of the 40 something plus crowd, alas not for everyone, again
pick the plan that works for you and don't be afraid to experiment
with these little side ideas, but stay the course.
This Doesn't mean to be a glutinous person.
Remember the Ben Franklins virtues of life take note of #1 and #9,
Temperance and Moderation.
I maintain that you need to nourish your body and keep your
metabolic engine (muscles) running all the time, slowing metabolism
causes the body to hoard fat and burn muscle.
A dyslexic way of looking at it for sure.

Beginning at age 30, the body naturally starts to lose 3–5% of muscle
mass per decade, this is our metabolic engine losing steam!

After 35 years of age - MEN lose about a pound of muscle a year.
After 35 years of age – Women gain a pound of cellular FAT weight
a year.

Skip a workout Don't skip a meal

Now I believe this happens mostly if we don't nourish the body with quality nutrition and exercise.

Many have the distorted idea of a healthy diet is eat less and workout more.. bzzzzzzz wrong answer!
This is also known as "starvation mode." If you're waiting too long to eat in the morning or in between meals, your metabolism can slow, which encourages your body to store calories as FAT instead of using them for energy. Get to know your sweet spot, oops wrong analogy, if you get to know your body the process gets so much easier, what We don't want is the evil FAT Lord of Darkness!

"Lord Sarcopenia" -Sarcopenia meaning : a syndrome characterized by progressive and generalized loss of skeletal muscle mass and this generally happens when someone gets older and does less physical activity..
 So Lets not go there, keep moving!

Declaration: Put your Hand on your Heart and say:

"Good results begin with GOOD choices."

CODE: EIGHT

Fuel the Engine – Whey Cool

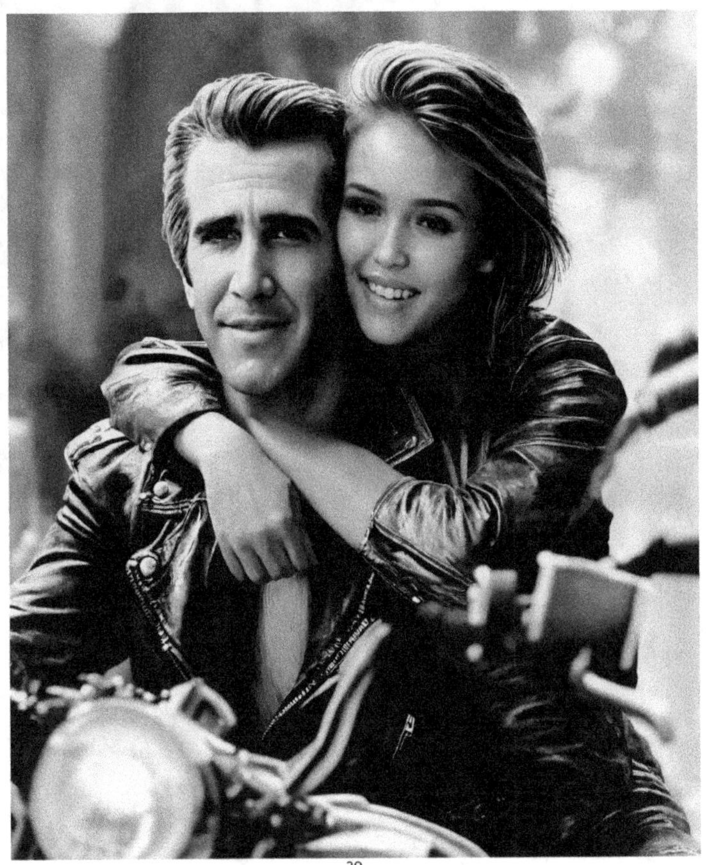

Fuel the Engine whey cool

CRACKING THE FAT CODE

Fuel the Engine - Whey Cool

A great Segway to my favorite topic – PROTEIN!
Increase protein do not skimp. Protein Protein Protein.
Over the years of training individuals Men and Women there really
is no difference when it comes to protein.

Men and Women both must feed and replenish the protein daily if
you watch the elderly they skimp on protein all the time.
We need between .5 grams to 1.0 gram per lean bodyweight
depending on activities. so if a person wants to maintain their muscle
on a 150 pound frame 75 to 150 grams of protein requirement daily.

Amino Acids are the building blocks of protein, there are
approximately 200 thousand chemical reactions that needs an amino
acid to do its function. There is alot going on in our body every
second of every day.
By days end we tend to rob Peter to pay Paul with our reserves and
then there is nothing left for building back our muscle tissue.
Not only that certain amino acids are needed to help you get to sleep
and repair, tryptophan and glycine to name a few.
Your Muscles are your metabolic engine that in turn burns calories
to fuel the engine!

…what is the number one metabolic burning calorie burning food?
PROTEIN - High protein foods…with adopting this Code there will
be overall, less abdominal fat, more satiety, and an increased
metabolic function.
Whey more muscle, Whey less weight, WHEY COOL!

Fuel the Engine whey cool

Protein is one of my forte's, my wheelhouse if you will.
 In the 1990s and beyond I sold a ton of protein shakes and other
sport supplements when I was working for a nutraceutical company
out of Toronto to health food stores across southwestern Ontario.
Constantly helping athletes gain lean muscle and helping women and
men lose that unwanted weight as they got ready for the beach
season, sport training or that upcoming wedding.

Doing protein demos at several health food stores was a weekly
endeavor for me. Sharing my sports knowledge, shake recipes and
knowledge of how adding a shake or two a day could help them get
to their wellness goals.Abundantly fun times in those days and
getting a high-quality protein shake is paramount.
 All proteins are not created equal and it's the extras that do more
harm then good!
 The garbage given to seniors is a disgrace ,you know the ready to
drink (RTD's) the ones in a can or a Tetra box these are horrid.
 This type of protein is at the bottom of the barrel and they don't
even give to rats when testing, no kidding!
 Wit sugars that shouldn't be in the protein products whatsoever.
Quite honestly the baby formulas are just as bad, for years I have
told, mother's to be and young mothers to make their own formula
with high quality protein, minerals and EFA's (good Fat).

 It doesn't take much more effort to do this, much better for the baby
and saves you money to boot.

CRACKING THE FAT CODE

When looking at a protein on the label it should show the **micro fractions** secondly be an isolate protein powder of a undenatured source.
The Protein should have a **high alpha content of 20% or more** just remember ALPHA as first or the prime one, the most important one!

Alpha-Lactalbumin is a protein fraction proven to offer superior health benefits including faster growth and repair of muscle tissue, stronger immune function. Alpha-lactalbumin as a protein source increases blood tryptophan levels, which promotes the synthesis and availability of serotonin in the brain. Alpha-lactalbumin provides 48 mg of cysteine per gram of protein.
Cysteine (amino acid) is the direct precursor to the antioxidant glutathione.
the specific effects of alpha-lactalbumin on the gut are in part from the bioactive peptides from the unique tryptophan and cysteine combination.
A ton of research has been done with glutathione and High Alpha whey and its amazing help combating against different diseases including cancer.

I won't go in depth here on this awesome subject, there are many resources on the Net to help you find your quality whey protein sources that work for your lifestyle, I will be coming out with a book completely about protein soon, so stay Tuned....
My favorite Protein shakes you can check out in the CODE 31 on supplements.

Declaration: Put your Hand on your Heart and say:

" My Body is nourished with the highest quality protein available"

Fuel the Engine whey cool

CODE: NINE

WATER we doing!

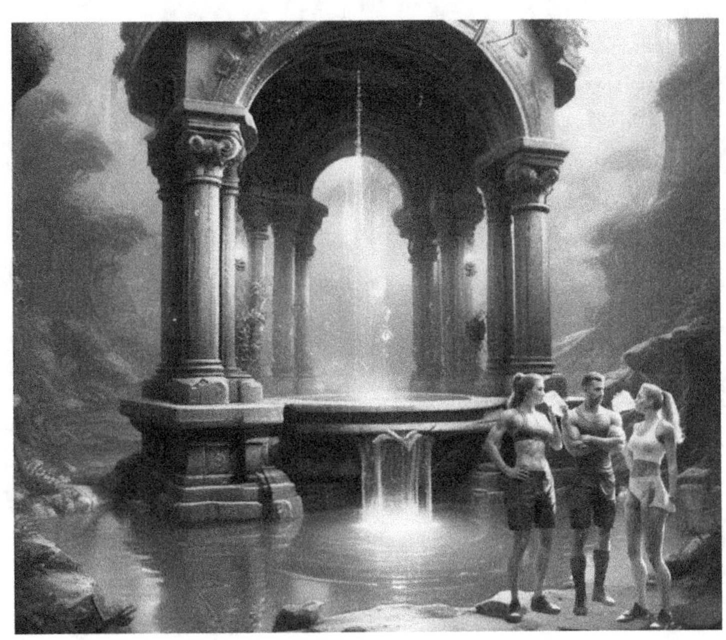

WATER we doing!

CRACKING THE FAT CODE

Water We Doing

WATER: So much is said about water this is a BIG topic and so many people fluff it off!

Lack of Water, dehydration and the importance of Quality H2O

"many degenerative diseases and other illnesses were simply the result of dehydration" - Dr. Fereydoon Batmanghelidj

Constipation for instance is most often the result of not drinking enough WATER and eating enough high fibre foods.

We will talk fibre in CODE 23.

Get into the habit of drinking plenty of quality water throughout the day make sure its quality water.

Studies have shown that drinking as little has 500ml (about 17 ounces) of water can boost your metabolism by up to 30%.

Muscles are 75% water, the human body is approximately 70% water, our blood is 83% water
we need to keep our WATER intake UP!

Drinking adequate amount of water is a must.
 I hear so many people say they don't drink enough and others say they don't like water not drinking water will lead to many illnesses down the road.
 I would guess for the most part the people that say they don't like water have had a bad experience with a a subpar source of water not to like it ,really its like saying you hate 70% of yourself.

 It absolutely must be quality water and when detoxifying even more important!

Water throughout the day will help flush the toxins out of the fat cells.
 We need on average .55 oz. per pound of body weight of H20 daily (more when exercising or vigorous activities).

WATER we doing!

TAP WATER -

Lets talk about Tap Water - tap water is known to have toxins because of the lack of filtration, so the epidemic of estrogen dominance is largely because of **Tap water.**
 90% of well water also because of the runoffs and it doesn't matter how deep the well is, it really doesn't unless your in a blue zone in the tropics.
Both Federal, State and Provincial governments in North America admit there is a Huge problem.

NEXT - Trihalomethanes (THMs) the result of a reaction between the chlorine used for disinfecting tap water and natural organic matter in the water.
At elevated levels EVERYWHERE in towns and cities.
THMs have been associated negative health effects over 36 known cancers and adverse reproductive outcomes.
So much research documented you just can't ignore this anymore! We are constantly informing people, from the front door of your home inward is your responsibility keep your family healthy.

 Take the initiative to protect and take care of yourself and your loved ones, get a a Quality whole home filtration system.

CRACKING THE FAT CODE

A great short video to show what is in the water is found at
arcradio.net called h2oh!
A video about asbestos in the water supply across North America
video found on youtube
called "something in the water" W5 investigation.

When I do lectures, I always include the water crisis I just have to its
not fear mongering yet since this is such a titanic sized issue in health
and Wellness it needs to be!

..We have become the "Water POLICE" over the last 30 years,
people have nick named Us this as we lecture on this to every client
and customer's since the late 1990's!

Again We humans are 70% water and no coincidence the earth is
70% water so our health is dictated by 70% of the type of water we
ingest?
Sounds about right I would have to bet strong that this is quite
possibly true.
I am a solution guy so always show the solutions to incorporate in
our lives and the lives of our community and loved ones, water being
a pivotal one in our health and well-being.
I do unearth numerous debates with country folk and farmers trying
to convince me that they have a well and in defiance claiming its
deep and the best water and there is nothing wrong with their water!

 WELL (pun intended) I beg to differ and if they do a deep dive into
all that's in the water, they will change their mind. Our own
provincial and federal government state on their websites that well
water **is contaminated** and they even go through the various
contaminants.
Alleviate the problem and get a filtration system best suited for the
environment you live then the issue is resolved.

WATER we doing!

Healthy water not just so called "safe" water. I work closely with two companies out of Windsor, Ontario that provide all of the solutions pertaining to "clean and healthy Water", to drink and shower in.
choices4water and aerusofwindsor.

If you talk to your municipality, they will call the water safe. I always retaliate with ,"Safe compared to what?!

 They have allowable amounts of substances in the water , would you like to ingest 300 to 2000 chemical of a small allowable amount and be ok with it?
If given the choice would you rather not have any of these substances in your water supply? You know the cancer causing substances, endocrine disruptors, microplastics, asbestos fibers, and the undigested pharmaceuticals that the subpar filtration systems can't handle?
This is what the government and municipalities call safe! So drink with, cook with and shower with **healthy water** not safe water.
Cheers!

A NEW HOPE in the Universe – Hydrogen?
 Hydrogen the most abundant element in the Universe now with much focus on hydrogen water and the Health of our Cells.
 Hydrogen, or H1, is the lightest element in the periodic table. In nature, hydrogen atoms tend to bond with other atoms. For example, when two hydrogen atoms bond, they form molecular hydrogen or H2. When H2 bonds with a single oxygen atom, this becomes water – commonly known as H2O.
So after you achieve Healthy systems in your home you just may want to kick it up a notch, "Bam", as Emeril use to holler on his cooking show.
 I find this upgrade in drinking water is a must in the pantry.

CRACKING THE FAT CODE

H2 or Hydrogen water has been shown to decrease inflammation, boost athletic performance, and even support slowing the aging process.

Furthermore articles in pubMed the enhanced H2 water eliminates fine particles from the lungs and blood by enhancing phagocytic activity (meaning the cells can help protect or eliminate infectious and non-infectious environmental particles from them)

Presently a breakthrough in this area of hydration science is quite impressive with tremendous upsides. Studies at Johns Hopkins University revealed a new way for water to quickly enter cells, helping us reach more advanced hydration that improves our bodies' ability to burn fat.

You will most likely hear the word AQUAPORINS more and more in articles and water research ahead.

 - Aquaporins (AQP) are integral membrane proteins that serve as channels in the transfer of water, and in some cases, small solutes (component of a solution) across the membrane.

All in all it's safe to say Hydrogen-infused water - "H2" is gaining popularity. Hydrogen-infused water, or "H2" is gaining popularity

I must caution you need to start with high quality H2O from reverse osmosis or distilled a it should additionally the water should be slightly alkaline 7.2 to 7.4 pH and then go through the process of H2 infusing. If not utilizing high quality H2O, aka Healthy Water using just tap water can be quite destructive with an unknown amount of chemicals, pharmaceuticals, chlorine and fluoride. You will be shuttling that toxic soup harmful to the human body into the cells more readily, kinda BAD idea!

WATER we doing!

CODE: TEN

Get the PLUNGER

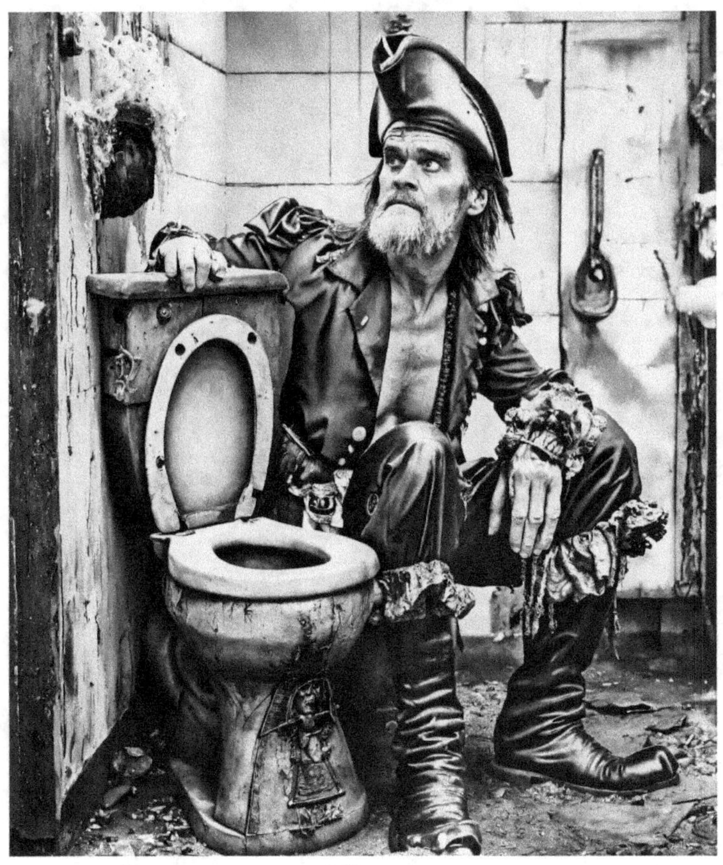

Get the PLUNGER

CRACKING THE FAT CODE

Get the PLUNGER

-Cleansing: The body needs a cleanse and done only with quality cleanses and must be done with high quality H2O - there are many cleanses on the market unfortunately many of these cleanse systems have harsh ingredients that can irritate the intestinal wall causing more harm than good. Do yourself a favor get a quality cleanse kit! Back to FAT cells here's the inside scoop they hold our toxins and the more toxins we have the more our fat cells increase in size (a fat cell can expand 1,000 times its size).

Doing a cleanse will help flush the toxins and help you lose your unwanted excess garbag eout of the FAT cells hence in doing so shrinking the fat cells, a twofer!

 Are you Regular – are you having at least one bowl movement a day if not STOP - no cleansing kits yet! you have to start there and must Get Regular with your bowel movements!

POOP Tuesdays

 - what is a normal bowel movement once or twice a week or once or twice a day what makes more sense to you?

On our old radio show we used to have a special guest a colon therapist and naturopathic Doctor. Every Tuesday all we talked about was digestive care and the importance of a proper bowel movement.

 So wE well, kinda me being a bit of joker, called it "poop Tuesday" and it stuck..oops bad pun.

So, the END point to this is If you're gonna try to detoxify the body you have to make sure you have proper bowel movements first this is key and must be addressed.

Getting regular means more water (quality water) moreover getting some supplement products that help with proper bowel movements. Natural products of course but nothing harsh.

Get the PLUNGER

We are meant to evacuate the toxins daily and best after every meal,
if your health provider is saying going 3 times a week is ok its just
you and how you are well bzzzzz WRONG! Sorry they are sadly
mistaken that is not how the human body works.
You must get to at least one bowel movement a Day. Every single
mammal on this planet eliminates daily and We are no different.
 Go into the memory banks and think. Here's a question have you
ever needed to go to the restroom/bathroom, you entered and there
is this awful stench Woo Weee, YUCK we all have been there you
know exactly what it is too! but hey there's curiosity so you open the
stall door and the toilet was not flushed and good LORD whatever
was deposited and evacuated from another entity is still there!! As
Gomer Pile would phrase "Golly", "Sur-prise, Sur-prise,
SURPRISE!"
So.. How long was the "Offering" in the porcelain throne? An hour a
day either way YA the vile stench frickin REEKS!
Ok you get the picture so now lets put this in perspective of YOU.
 Think about this with YOU the foods eaten the past 24 hours are
digesting butt,(pun intended), has nowhere to go so the excrement
(the toxins) just stay put and ferment in your body.
Do you really think this is a good idea and normal for fermented
garbage to collect inside you for days?
Absolutely NOT, so number one - GET REGULAR before moving
on to a cleanse, check the fibre CODE 23 for more on this as well as
the Cleanse CODE 14 !
Some Supplements I will suggest that will help the process and do so
without harm or irritation. The first I will mention is try a high-
quality magnesium in the BIS glycinate or citrate form and finding
your threshold.
Doctor Linus Pauling came up with the threshold method where let's
say your threshold is 1000 milligrams of magnesium. Meaning this is
where you get really loose stools, THAT's your threshold. Now back
up your magnesium intake to to 900 milligrams or 800 milligrams
and this would be your safe zone.

CRACKING THE FAT CODE

You can apply this to a lot of supplements, this a great way get to know your Body internally.

Secondly is to increase your fibre intake refer the the Fibre CODE23

Thirdly, a quality elimination product possibly from our good friends from Healthology here's what they say:

We should aim to have at least one easy-to-pass, fully evacuated bowel movement per day. If you are having infrequent, difficult-to-pass, or incompletely evacuated bowel movements, then you're likely experiencing constipation. The causes of constipation are many, with dehydration, inflammation in the gut, unhealthy gut flora, stress, low-fibre diet, and a slow metabolism being common factors

The wave-like contractions and relaxations of muscles that move stool through the bowel is called peristalsis, and diminished peristaltic function can lead to constipation.

When stool sits in the colon for a long period of time, it re-absorbs too much water, making the stool dry, hard, and difficult to pass.

Check out their product in the supplement Code 31 section.

There are other supplements you can use that can help you become regular a proper BM but I would stay away from the harsh products on the market and that includes the orange coloured bottle at the local pharmacy.

Check out the supplement chapter for a few of my favorites that have helped a lot of clients and customers over the years.

Declaration: Put your Hand on your Heart and say:

" I Let GO, Rather than Hold ON."

Get the PLUNGER

CODE: ELEVEN

TAPIN to your Temple

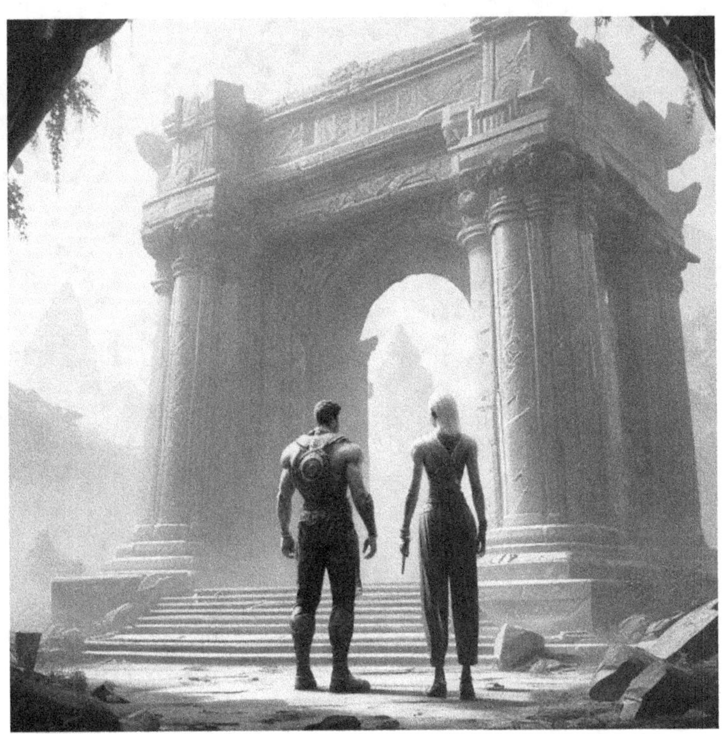

TAPIN to your Temple

CRACKING THE FAT CODE

TAPIN to your Temple

"Get your Ass in shape – your Health is your Wealth"
- Miami Multi Millionaire.

Being interviewed by a well known youtuber the first thing out of the fit 40 something millionaires' mouth was the above Statement.

 This is so true you can't take your wealth with you to your grave but you can take with you a vibrant and healthy body. More people are living longer but merely living unhealthy longer, that sucks.

Exercising: Ya I know I am using the **E** word...Don't blow it off! We were meant to move but yes we can over do it as well. You don't have to train like an Olympian but being a coach potato is unhealthy and decreases your energy levels sizably including your waist.

Move it, get a personal trainer, join a class, whatever suits you and your situation.

Move that body, like a ship in the harbor if the ship(your body) doesn't move it rusts and develops barnacles our barnacles being bulkier volumized fat cells, inflammation and the like.

Take the Time:

Just a 30 minute workout from your 1440 minutes of the day.

 4 times a week(that's only 120 minutes a week) of your 10,080 minutes of the week.

In three months that is only 1548 minutes of the 3 month 130,032 minutes.

Just those 120 minutes a week will help you get to where you need to be in three months.

 We're all given 24 hours a day or 14140 minutes ...

There is no excuse, we all have the same amount of time you just have to take the TIME.

Make it a good habit in your LIFE your body and mind will thank you for it ....I think you already know that!

Exercise changes how fat tissue looks and behaves.
 Study from
- October 12, 2022 at the University of Michigan -
    Exercise can modify FAT tissue in ways that improve health even without weight loss
The study aimed to better understand the effects of exercise on metabolic health in people with obesity. Thirty-six adults with obesity were placed into either a moderate-intensity exercise group (45 minutes, 70% of maximum heart rate) or a high-intensity exercise group (10 one-minute intervals at 90% maximum heart rate interspersed with 60 seconds of low-intensity active recovery).

Blood samples and biopsies of abdominal fat were collected the day after the 12-week sessions ended and again three days later.

 There was no exercise between these tests. Results for both exercise groups showed several structural changes in fat tissue, including slightly smaller fat cells and more of them, increased collagen type, increased capillary density, and changes in proteins that regulate body fat remodeling.

Horowitz said many of the changes in factors regulating body fat remodeling seen one day after exercise were no longer significant on day 4 of testing, and this underscores the importance of regular, sustained exercise.
Improvements disappeared when exercise stopped.

CRACKING THE FAT CODE

We eat, breathe, drink (water) everyday…we need to move that body everyday!

Many adaptations to exercise training are effective in enabling a person to exercise longer or harder, Horowitz said.

"However, most of the benefits of exercise that improve metabolic health in people at risk for metabolic health complications or those who have metabolic disease stems from the response to each exercise session.

These responses to exercise are relatively short-lived, often lasting only a few days at most," he said. "This is one of the big reasons why it is so important to be physically active most days."

Just going for a stroll? There's nothing wrong with walking it is a form of low impact to moderate intense workout it has benefits with few risks.

Experts say that you need about 8 kilometers or five miles a day for you to get in shape. To speed up the process this is my suggestion:

Just adding some squats (resistance exercise) just your bodyweight or with light weights five sets of 10 before walking will turn on your metabolic engine BIG TIME before you start your walk the benefits will be much more profound.

When doing squats the most important thing is to execute the movement with strict form and modify it depending on your capabilities.

I've heard this so often" oh I'm just gonna start jogging and then I'll start doing weights in a few weeks" this is an outdated and old paradigm.

Do them Both for the best benefit!

Resistance training changes the way fat cells operate and triggers the fat-burning process throughout our bodies.

Can exercise activate brown fat?

Exercise activates the sympathetic nerve, (responsible for the fight or flight response), boosting the activity of brown fat, improving heat production, and regulating the metabolism of sugar and FAT. Thus amplifying your metabolism burning calories, shrinking FAT cells, and hey LOOK the jeans are fitting better now.

Dissolving a Myth

No you won't get Big and Bulky by lifting weights or doing resistance training. Resistance builds a lean body(not bulky) and boosts your metabolism, the end.

For women this is very True. First women don't have the testosterone that men have for huge muscles in fact women have around 20% less muscle mass then a man.

Secondly have you seen many women at an "all you can eat" buffet? Not many, the patrons are mostly all men. A woman's daily calorie intake is generally much less then the caloric intake of a mans.

As far as Bulking Up goes its how a man or women lifts meaning the amount of weight on a device to do your exercises.

An example are squats the "king of exercises" my opinion.

We should all do squats as one of my mentors Dr. Michael Colgan says ",your legs are like two Doctors, use them and move them".

 The weight makes the difference here if your doing 50 pounds on the barbell or 2-25 pound dumbbells' and perform the movements your not getting bulky, your getting stronger and tone.

If you compound each set putting more loads each time of 250, 300, to 400 pounds on the Bar well of course your getting bigger muscles.

Most woman its safe to say are not powerlifters and generally most men aren't eithers so the BULK idea just doesn't happen easily, its actually quite hard for most.

Don't be intimidated or think your going to look like the incredible HULK that's a BIG NO.

Weight lifting/resistance training helps you tone and increase your health and that's the fact Jack, so happy lifting

The Windfall of weights
Physical and cognitive benefits of resistance training include:
Improved muscle strength and body toning, protects the joints from injury, better flexibility and balance.
Assists with preventing cognitive decline, accelerates stamina, and controlling heart disease, diabetes, back pain and other chronic conditions.
 Resistance training also supports your posture as well increases your bone density.
 Enhances better sleep, a sense of well-being, hence better mood and more
self-confidence!
Just a few positive things eh?
Anaerobic exercise - Weight Training
Anaerobic exercise is a type of exercise that breaks down glucose in the body without using oxygen; anaerobic means "without oxygen."
I'm a big believer in resistance training, (anaerobic training) –
From my own experiences and countless clients that I worked with I place confidence in resistance training with mindful aerobic activities.
 You will become much more lean then just going for a little jog around the neighborhood block or on a treadmill reading a magazine or watching the news. Furthermore, in doing this later activity you are not engaging your brain body connection (Mindful workout).
If you're gonna watch the news watch the news, if you're gonna read a book then read a book aside from that if your going to train your body then train optimally, utilize your mind and body together time for some Mindfulness workouts!
In doing this you will burn noticeably more calories.
Many studies point out Resistance training fires up your metabolic rate then continues throughout the day and even when you sleep.

TAPIN to your Temple

The Lactic Acid dilemma -
        When you work your muscles to a point that they're not used
to your body creates a substance called lactic acid most people think
that lactic acid is a bad thing but it's actually a good thing.
Lactic acid keeps your muscles flexing and helps you get those few
extra reps in.

Lactic acid actually stimulates testosterone and GH - growth
hormone production and YES this is good for both men and women
testosterone and Growth Hormone stimulate repair and boost your
metabolism even more!
The takeaway…simple…The Body and Mind need to be connected
for optimal results they are your twin flames for metabolic harmony.
If you're going to do some aerobic training on a treadmill, stepper a
jog around the block couple it with first doing some resistance
training before you go.

Time to Tap IN and optimize your body TEMPLE!

Declaration: Put your Hand on your Heart and say:

" I am now Willing to Change my Whole LIFE."

CODE: TWELVE

The TEMPLE of DOOM

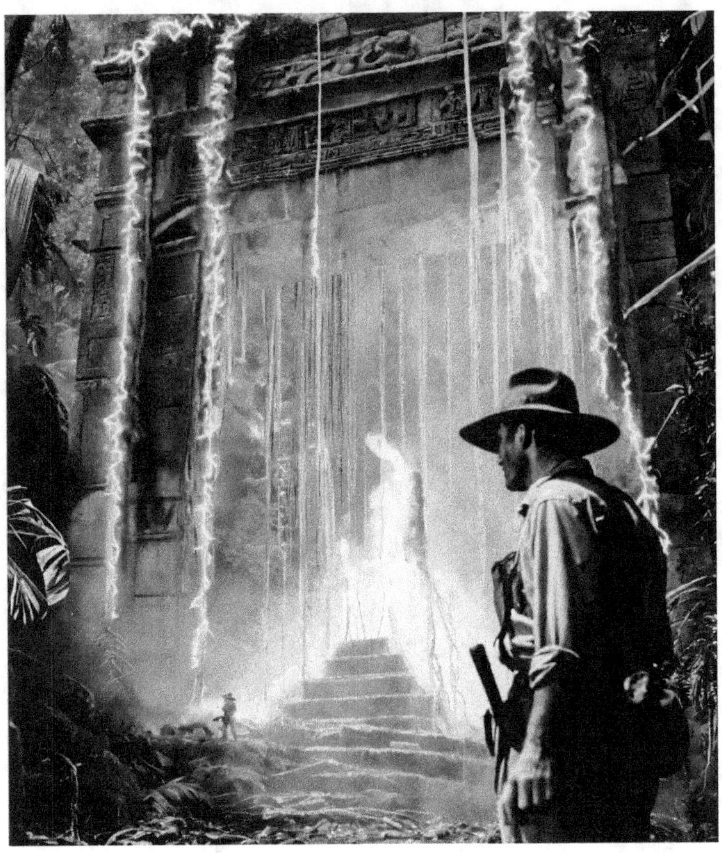

The Temple of DOOM

CRACKING THE FAT CODE

The Temple of DOOM

I'm Doomed my Moms FAT and my Dad is More FAT - I Can't WIN!

Genetics, yep that's the Ol' Storyline.

Don't let the 3% dictate your life and keep you in a victim mentality! I hear the victims all the time say ...." I don't have the genetics" or "its my genetics that's why I am FAT, my mother and father are both obese."

.I call this the kingdom of the blah, blah, blahs .. It reminds me of one of my childhood books "The Blah" – by Jack Kent , Morale of the story don't be bullied by BIG Brother, and they LIE.

Genetics only play into 3 % that's IT! 3 percent of the total figure with regards to the human body.

You have 97% or more to play with (epigenetics) so don't even go there this is the loser mentality the victim mentality, I may get some haters out there now on this ,sorry truth hurts.

You are in the drive seat, now take control and get out ofthe temple of Doom.

Epigenetics means above the (jeans- maybe it should say beneath?) Above the Genes meaning you have control over your genetic potential. Your in control over what you do on a daily basis you have the POWER ,and since we turn over billions of cells daily what you do daily dictates the Petri dish you lived in yesterday, the one your in today and also tomorrow.

Time for A COOL Change -little River Band – I can hear the lyrics from the song as I write this. Great lyric here: "there's lots of those friendly people, They're showing me ways to go but I never want to lose their inspiration, Time for a COOL Change!"

Enough of a little genetic debris, move to a NEW COOL Paradigm!

Declaration: Put your Hand on your Heart and say:

" I Now Value My Body."

The Temple of DOOM

CODE: THIRTEEN

You have the POWER

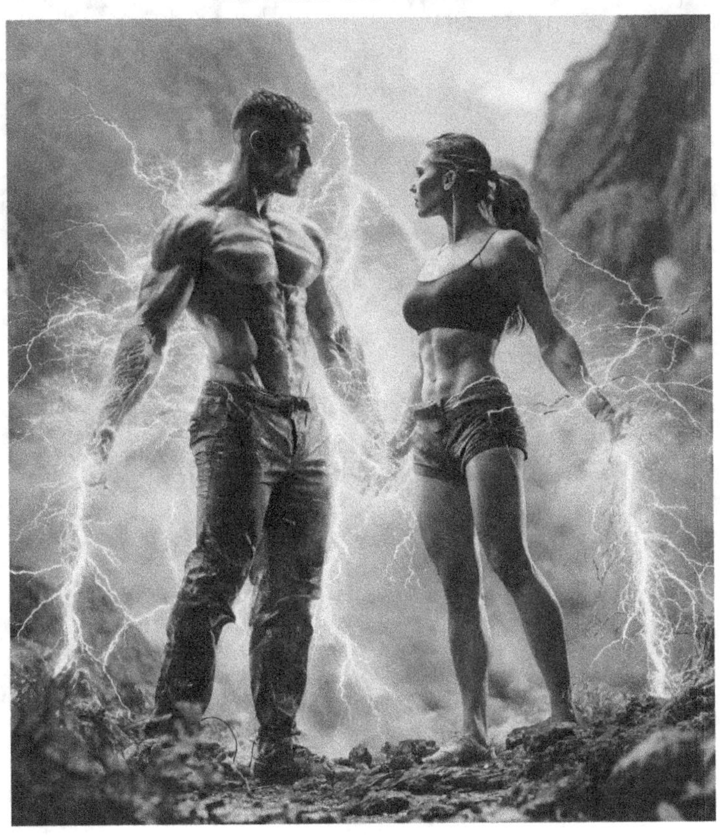

You have the POWER

CRACKING THE FAT CODE

EPIGENETICS (above your genes)
YES this puts you in the driver seat , you are in control.
 In control of your destiny!
Rise UP, you and only you have the POWER to change
no-one else … it all starts and ends with YOU!
We were taught if Gramma has heart disease, then its passed down
to Mom therefore Mom will have heart disease and so guess what
mom passed it to you and presto you will have heart disease..
Oh ya and don't forget there is nothing you can Do about it, says
main stream medical.
Hear this before from the white coats perhaps, It's in the family and
its your genetic destiny…

I can Darth Vader saying – "come join Me on the Dark Side of the
FORCE!"
I can hear the buzzer again bzzzzzzzzzzzzzzzzzzzzzzzz - WRONG!
You don't Have to go to the Dark side!
The Dark lord of genetics is partially correct, a minuscule 3% correct
that puny genetic weakness that micro part of the dark side doesn't
have to be an issue ever in your life! It is a tiny little factor that's it.

Its a victim mentality, I say Hogwash and its B.S. (bad science) you
can do something, more than something you can DO all of the
things and situations in your petri dish of your LIFE.
Epigenetically your behaviors and environment can cause changes
that affect the way your genes work. Dissimilar to genetic changes,
epigenetic changes are reversible and do not change your DNA
sequence, they can however change the way your body reads a DNA
sequence. You are in the driver Seat!

You have the POWER

The NOW and The Future
Your Petri Dish which is the environment 97% are Up to YOU!

Your life your body and mind, there is no lack or victimization there
only if you let it be that way..

YOU are in control of everything, now isn't that's EMPOWERING!

As you read and adopt all of these CODES that in itself will in fact
put you in the Drivers seat.
It will champion your POWER and Optimize your LIFE experience
and bolster changes in the Environment in which you live.

Declaration: Put your Hand on your Heart and say:

"I Now take Full responsibly for MY LIFE!"

CODE: FOURTEEN

Lucky #7

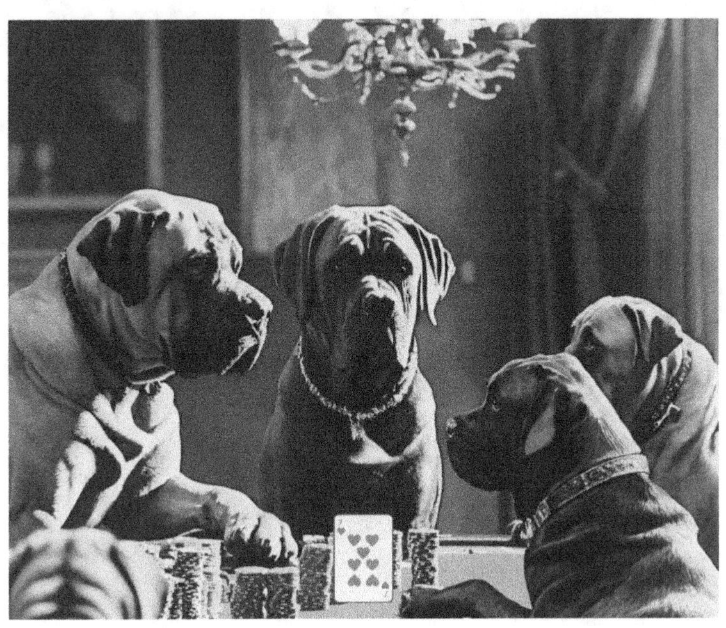

Lucky#7

Lucky # 7

The Seven channels of elimination

Many conventional people will say that we can detoxify the body without any help, the body will do everything it needs to do.

It's unfortunate the medical world will poopoo (kinda pun intended) any alternative way to address the body detox strategies that many people use to keep in Optimal Health and I have seen it work for the last 30 plus years right before my eyes, Nature Provides!

I am here to 100% disagree with those of the conventional thinking.

We do not live in the garden of Eden. its fact however that we do live in a toxic world these days.

Cleansing and detoxification are totally essential for healing the digestive tract and restoring them to prime function.

The body has several ways for detoxification

The Lucky # 7- lets explore

#1 THE LUNGS: They expel toxins with every breath and as you know we breathe out is carbon dioxide being a byproduct of respiration and we breathe in oxygen.

With every breath we take we expel toxins but also inhale toxins the severity depending where you are living and breathing kind of a catch 22.

#2 THE LIVER: the general manager of the detoxification systems in our body.

We are in a Toxic world researchers believe because of the burden placed on the liver it can't keep up and because of this it contributes to many chronic difficulties.

Chronic fatigue, high cholesterol, IBS, cognitive difficulties, and high blood pressure are because of the excess burden placed on the Liver.

#3 THE KIDNEYS: our kidneys filter oak water-soluble wastes and these waste our from the blood that flows from the liver they are stored in the bladder and then eliminate it through our urine.

#4 THE BLOOD: Key transportation system bringing nutrients to the cells and also flushing away the toxins from the cells.

 #5 THE LYMPH: - a clear fluid filled with immune cells called lymphocytes this watery fluid provides nutrients to cells and tissues throughout the body to protect the body from a possible foreign invasion of bacteria ,viruses and cancer cells.

#6 THE SKIN: our biggest organ of the body it's kind of our armor keeping toxins from entering the body and because of it being our biggest organ it eliminates more waste than the colon and the kidneys combined

#7 THE COLON the end of the line the final destination the end point before toxins are eliminated
 There's a lot of colon cancer out there This is why proper bowel movements daily must happen.
Many people go to a colon therapist and have a colon cleanse, and this is well and good, what about the rest of the digestive system and all those other channels of elimination?
 If you don't address the other six channels, then you put a ton of pressure pun intended on your colon, if you work with all of them together then you may never have to do a colon cleanse.
 I never have and not to say that I ever will but there is no need to as of right now due to the care I've taken on all of the channels of elimination.
 In doing so I've helped my body maintain a clean Petri dish AKA my epigenetic environment as much as possible while following all of the CODES in this book.

CRACKING THE FAT CODE

The BEST CLEANSE I know
- My favorite story:

The story of Rene Caisse, This brave and courageous woman
helped over 5000 people that were sent home what terminal cancer to
die. These 5000 people lived!
This miraculous herbal blend in a Herbal TEA form was
administered by this nurse in Bracebridge, Ontario, Canada. This
Flor-Essence product is my all time favorite product for helping the
body with cleansing and helps with all those seven channels of
elimination.
I am sharing this story because it doesn't get told enough and is dear
to my heart as my wife had the opportunity to meet Elaine
Alexander but I am getting a head a little bit so.....

Back to the Origins – In 1922, the Canadian nurse, Rene Caisse, was
given the names of eight different herbs by a woman she met in a
hospital who had originally been given them by an Ojibwa medicine
man.
Over the course of the next several decades, she worked out of her
clinic (in the Bracebridge Hotel) and with various doctors using the
eight herbs in various strengths and combinations.
Eventually she came up with two formulas. Rene and Dr. Brusch.
Dr. Charles Brusch, President John F. Kennedy's personal physician
decided to carry on using the original eight herbs in a formula that
they had developed in partnership.

This formula came to be known as Flor-Essence when it made its way to
 Flora Manufacturing after Rene Caisse had passed away and Dr. Brusch signed over its rights to Elaine Alexander, a radio broadcaster on health issues. Elaine brought this formula to Flora, based in British Columbia Canada.

That's the True story of Flor-Essence the END....
Alot of misinformation out in the world this is the correct information – Now its even hard to find any information about Elaine the go between and not to mention all of the documentation that showed results of the patients. Like a good Cleanse they were Eliminated!
Makes you go Hummmm?
Back to the Amazing Herbal TEA -

It is easy and can be done slowly and mildly or more aggressively if need be.
 This was made with a perfect combination the only ONE of its kind.

Declaration: Put your Hand on your Heart and say:

" I am now Conscious of everything I DO."

CODE: FIFTEEN

The YEAST Beast!

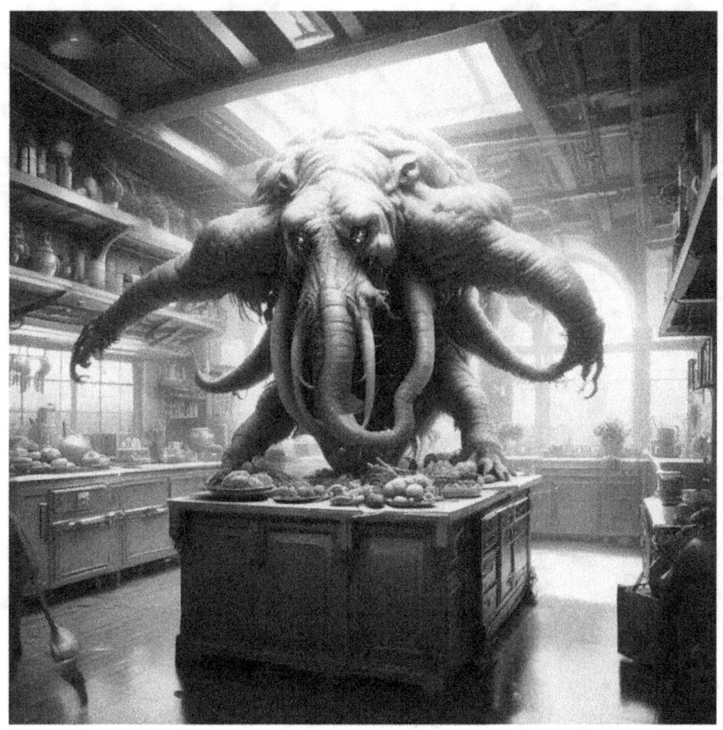

The YEAST Beast

THE YEAST BEAST!

- Candida overgrowth, Candida albicans (yeast).

Candida overgrowth can not only make you FAT, but also make it near impossible to shed those extra pounds.
If you find that you have been struggling with your weight and uncontrollable sugar for years, then you most likely have been misdiagnosed or undiagnosed.

The Candida conundrum - we dove into this topic of Candida quite a bit over the years on our radio show when we had Dr. Brenda Watson a colon therapist and a naturopathic Dr. On our show the following is information from a few of her books and from our talks on the "Wellness with Kim show."
According to Dr. Brenda Watson and her colleges -one of trillions of microscopic organisms present in the human digestive tract throughout the entire life cycle.
Candida albicans makes up nearly **75 percent of the body's immune system** and if that delicate balance of beneficial to harmful bacteria in the intestinal tract is disturbed, disease-causing microorganisms may be allowed to thrive and multiply.

In the case of Candida albicans, the destructive yeast will invade and damage the surrounding tissues, and in severe situations the overgrowth may spread to the bloodstream. This problem can be traced back to individual diet and lifestyle habits. These are the scenario's we learned on the radio shows and having experts in the field discuss the problems and the solutions to the imbalances.

The YEAST Beast

Among the most common of causes are from a bacterial imbalance in the gut many times due to stress, illness, the misuse or overuse of prescription antibiotics and acid-blocking drugs; the use of cortisone and other steroids. Overconsumption of sugar and refined carbohydrates; fluctuating hormone levels (common in women during PMS and pregnancy); and exposure to toxins such as mercury (typically from dental fillings), which kills the good bacteria that keep destructive yeast under control.
An effective natural yeast prevention program must first begin with necessary diet changes this can be remedied with proper nutritional foods and/or a possible candida cleanse.
Fibre and enzymes are essential when it comes to preventing yeast overgrowth. Taking digestive enzymes between meals can help break down Candida albicans by attacking its cell walls.
Too many people fail to add this to the regime and wonder why the protocol wasn't very successful, this is generally why this the case so please ADD the fibre and enzymes.
 On an empty stomach right before bed, take a multi-strain enzyme supplement that contains protease, cellulase, amylase, lipase, lactase and other plant-derived enzymes.
This big topic needs to be addressed getting your candida in order can be very difficult there are many candida diets on the web to follow. This shouldn't be taken lightly – remember Candida albicans makes up nearly 75 percent of the body's immune system.
So really this cleanse should be done at least once a year.
If there is a cell well-being practitioner close to where you live get a Cell Wellbeing Bio Hair Scan done this will give you the proper road map as to whether this is a priority or not.   cell-wellbeing.com

Declaration: Put your Hand on your Heart and say

" I am in touch with my physical Body, I am AWARE."

CODE: SIXTEEN

El Fuego

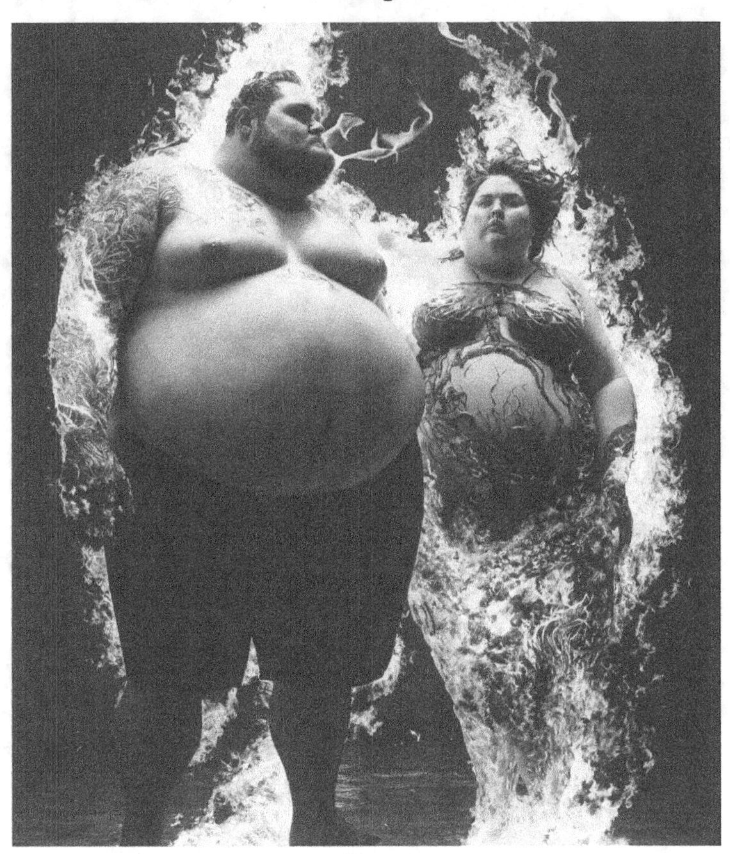

El Fuego

CRACKING THE FAT CODE

El Fuego - The FIRE

El Fuego, Inflammation

This is a whole book onto itself, and my close friend Brad king wrote a book on this very topic called *"Conquer Inflammation"*, showing how to put out the FIRES!
It has been shown that chronic, low-grade FAT tissue inflammation has long been associated with obesity.
 Chronic inflammation plays a prominent role in the development of weight gain much do to the inflammatory cytokines, markers that cause the inflammation like mediocre food choices.
The four main foods I disclose for clients to eliminate, even as little as a few weeks to see the difference, are anything related to: sugar, wheat, corn and dairy.
 - While inflammation is a natural process that has ensured our survival through generations, the relentless assaults of today's environment, stress, pollution, poor nutrition, and sleep, to name a few.
These all-trigger endless inflammatory responses that continuously harm your body-eventually leading to illness.
This is a major target, getting rid of the inflammation is key to helping other functions of the body do their job.

Manipulating many of the other Codes in this book will most certainly help rid the body of most inflammation.

Declaration: Put your Hand on your Heart and say:

" I let things happen by letting go of the Results."

El Fuego

CODE: SEVENTEEN

Creepshow

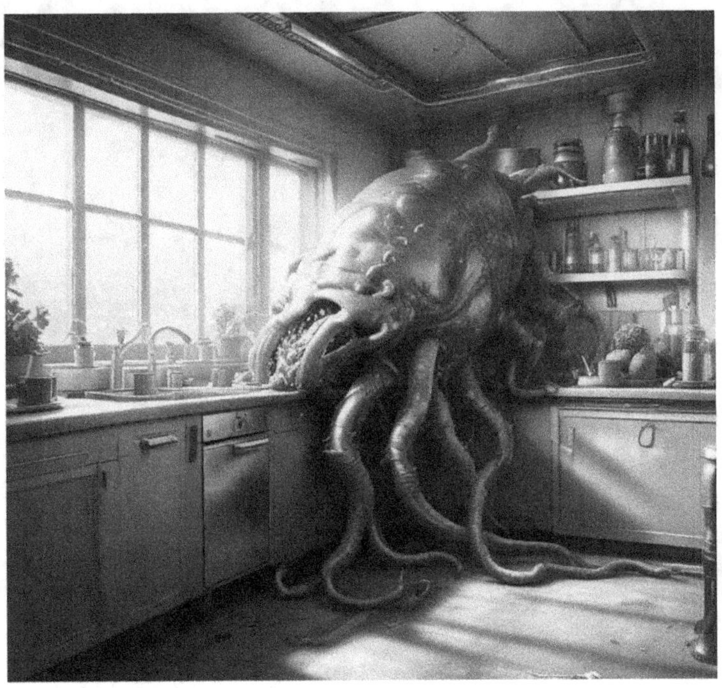

CreepShow

CRACKING THE FAT CODE

Creep show

Parasites – Oh No!

Well like it or not Humans have many and generally close to 300 parasitic worms and over 70 species of protozoa. So, they are a normal part of lif for Us even though it seems creepy.
Do you have pets? live on a farm? vacation in a different country?
We all do have parasites but when we pick up the wrong ones they can affect your mood, your well being, and can interfere your natural absorption of vitamins and minerals.
There are different ways to approach this from parasite cleanses to other natural ways to remove excess parasites.
 One is simply doing diatomaceous earth daily , do some research and follow their directions.
 Another is using AlliMax a bioactive stabilized form of Allicin from garlic it has the potency of 47 cloves of garlic with each capsule, so quite powerful without smelling like a dead corpse and vampires will assuredly stay away.
 I use this product habitually and the bonus is it helps alleviate viral and bacterial issues as well.
We do live on a small hobby farm so its just something we always stay ahead of and knock on wood I have never had excess creepy stuff..
 There is a protocol to use the AlliMax if utilized for removal of parasites. Check it out before commencing for optimal results.

Declaration: Put your Hand on your Heart and say:

"Wisdom is attained when Knowledge is Applied."

CreepShow

CODE: EIGHTEEN

Farmers feed Cities – Hero or Villain?

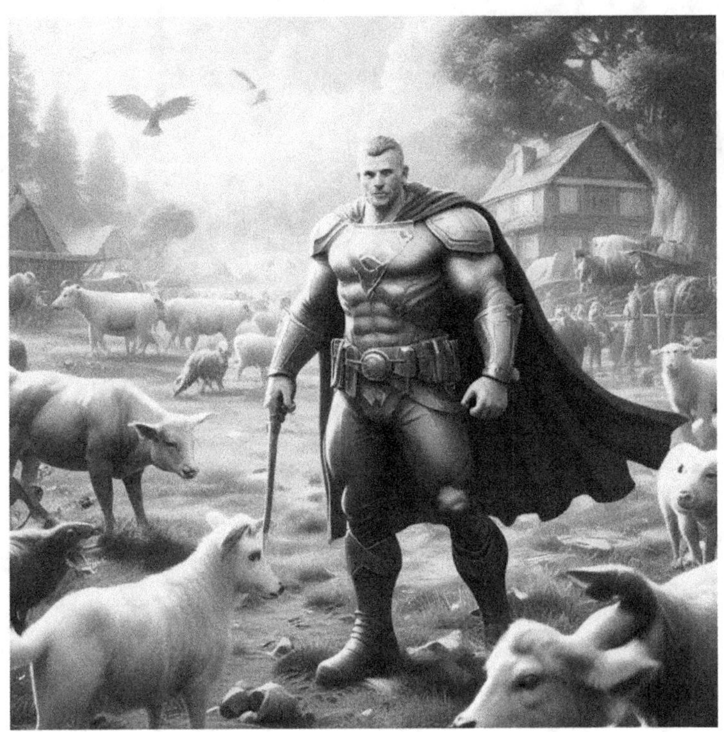

Farmers feed Cities - Hero or Villain?

CRACKING THE FAT CODE

Farmers, Hero or Villain?

"Farmers FEED Cities" - the Slogan
What are farmers feeding cities? That is the bigger question and we
need to take a hard look at the options to change! WE are receiving
and ingesting wrong food choices!
GMO's, MSG and other chemicals in the food, rancid Fats bad
vegetable fats .ie canola, artificial sweeteners and lots more. Watch a
great documentary called "OILING of AMERICA". This will give
you some insight!
I don't think I need to go into this too deeply we really should know
what we should eat and what we should eliminate going more for the
healthy choices. I call it the 80/20 Rule eat clean 80% of the time
indulge 20% I would say by the state of most people the numbers are
reversed, people have be misguided.
The processed foods the fried foods the white breads all the deserts
need to be put on hold or to a minimum.
NON-GMO does matter Don't eat GMO's don't buy into the
GMO's will save the world B.S. its killing the World if anything.
 There is so much compelling science to show what it does to the
human body and how GMO corn and other product's do make you
gain more weight its an epidemic.
 There are documentaries to watch on the subject: The Future of
Food, Oiling of America, GMO OMG, The World According to
Monsanto, and Genetic Roulette to name a few.
BIG-AGRA doesn't want to talk about any of this and doesn't want
you to think about it.
For those that want to look at the brighter future and some films to
show what can be done
Are : The Need To Grow, The Biggest Little Farm, and Kiss The
Ground, great documentaries for our regenerative future.
Conventional farmers don't want to talk about it and generally
poopoo the idea and get agitated when one brings up the subject.

Farmers feed Cities - Hero or Villain?

We need farmers to be Hero's again not the villainy that they have become because of the corruption of Big AGRA. Start to apply the regenerative principles to restore the soil and our FOOD and show their passion in what they have spent their lives in and to be the Hero once again.

In the meantime, find your local sources talk with the small hobby farms that are using these principles using no pesticides and feeding the soil so your food will be rich in nutrients.
There are plenty of heroes in the farming community adopting the regenerative farming practices and way of thinking.
The Top headliner or one of them for sure is a Hero Farmer, Joel Salatin.
I own a few of his books ,One called "Everything I want To Do Is Illegal."
Joel owns Polyface Farm a 550-acre farm where he pasture raises cattle and has the chickens swoop in behind and cleanup hence fertilizing the fields.

He is the One who made the "Chicken tractors" famous around the world and he is generally the #1 keynote speaker at holistic farming events across North America and beyond.
Another resource on YouTube is - OFF Grid with Doug & Stacy with their homesteading principles. This couple came from the city with no idea how to do off grid and farming. Now over a decade behind them they show how it can be done and have a ton of hints and ideas to share.

The Spice of life – and that's IT!

When using spices make sure it's just the spices and the herbs and that's it! I had to throw this into the mix cause people tend to forget this and forget about the **other ingredients**, many products hide the **other ingredients** under the heading spices so Beware!

CRACKING THE FAT CODE

Dr Doris Rapp MD, an environmental Doctor wrote the Book "Is This Your Child" and had a clinic set up to treat many with reactions to Food additives etc.
She was a wealth of knowledge a few videos are still roaming around the interweb while still on Youtube check out her videos.

Additives - anything with additives and you're not sure my motto is "when in doubt throw it out!"
There are pages of additives that are put into foods that you need to be aware of.
Many chemicals you can't even pronounce and if you can't you need to learn what those are some are for stability and emulsification some are for shelf life but most cause illness one bite at a time.
New research finds that those substances, which make ice cream creamy and salad dressings smooth, could also be making you FAT and keeping you FAT.
Generally if you can't pronounce it or spell it don't ingest it, do your research or the easier thing to do, just avoid it!
One that seems to be in more and more foods I will briefly explain is carrageenan there is a lot of controversy on this one if it's food grade they say it won't hurt or harm you.
From PUB-Med "Carrageenan in the Western diet may contribute to the development of diabetes and the effects of high fat consumption." Also "in a previous report, we identified exposure to the common food additive carrageenan as a cause of abnormal glucose tolerance and insulin resistance."
There are a ton of products that have carrageenan in them from soft tacos to creamers. I am seeing more and more of this garbage in products so for sure it must be cheap and they don't care, You need to take heed and Do this for YOU.

Farmers feed Cities - Hero or Villain?

   I for one would stay away from this as much as possible instead grab an alternative look for pectin or guar gum with less issues. I find anytime there is controversy and in doubt don't consume.

 There are a lot of healthy foods and alternatives We Just need to take the time to make sure we know what we are feeding our bodies! For FAT Burning go for **metabolic enhancing** FOODS and add these to your daily intake the internet is great but can be over whelming with contradictions everywhere. Stay on your Road to Wellness and pick and choose your daily intake wisely.
I kinda follow the Mediterranean way of eating and I modify it with items that are not generally on the diet like Hemp Hearts, it's quite clean and an easy to follow way to eat probably the most sustainable.
 I like the term lifestyle not DIET…who wants to DIE…it?
A few: Metabolic enhancing foods and combos to share:
HEMP HEARTS: We get our Hemp products from the Man that coined the term "Hemp Hearts" - Roger Snow from Alberta , his "Better then Organic" line of products are top notch. In Salsa (the hemp hearts thicken the salsa) – with organic (Non-GMO) corn chips enhanced with chia and hemp hearts, this a great snack/meal anytime of the day for anyone.
 In yogurt with Chia. Hemp with Oatmeal (beware of bad Oatmeal) or cereal – although most cereals are have TOO much crap in them including Folic Acid (synthetic Folate) which will cause many cellular disruptions. ALMONDS - EFA's - Healthy fatty acids and protein in almonds give the body a temporary metabolism kick. Enjoy 10 of each, whole almonds, some walnut, pecans, some peanuts mixed together as a nutritious snack.
I can't help it I Love My Nuts.. lol!

CRACKING THE FAT CODE

APPLES - spread almond butter on an apple
   I Love apples ,we planted five different heirloom organic varieties on our property and now we are able to harvest our own, so grateful!

Why Apples - An Apple contain pectin, a type of fiber that acts as a prebiotic in your gut microbiome which aids digestion also an apple has five grams of soluble fiber and remember one gram of fiber releases seven calories so a good choice for a snack. Apple skins have a rich source of quercetin a polyphenol an important group of antioxidants. The old saying "an apple a day keeps the doctor away" has much truth to it, again make it an organic apple of the heirloom variety if you can find it and enjoy.

SWEET POTATOES - contain both soluble and insoluble fiber
 -and yes we want more fiber so these are something to enjoy while getting to that personal weight.
They are a low glycemic food, so don't cause blood sugar spikes and crashes that can make you lack energy or prematurely hungry.

Nuts - Walnuts with omega-3 fatty acids, fiber, and plant-based proteins are a great snack to munch on and in addition a study showed walnuts appears to activate a brain area involved with impulse control.

EGGS - Yes, eggs can help you lose weight its how you prepare that counts, a complete high-quality protein source, because they contain all 9 essential amino acids. Be mindful on how you cook them.
There are SO many more foods to enjoy, always remember everything in moderation and of a high-quality Source – You Deserve IT!

Declaration: Put your Hand on your Heart and say:

"My Intuition Guides Me."

Farmers feed Cities - Hero or Villain?

CODE: NINETEEN

ACID Trip

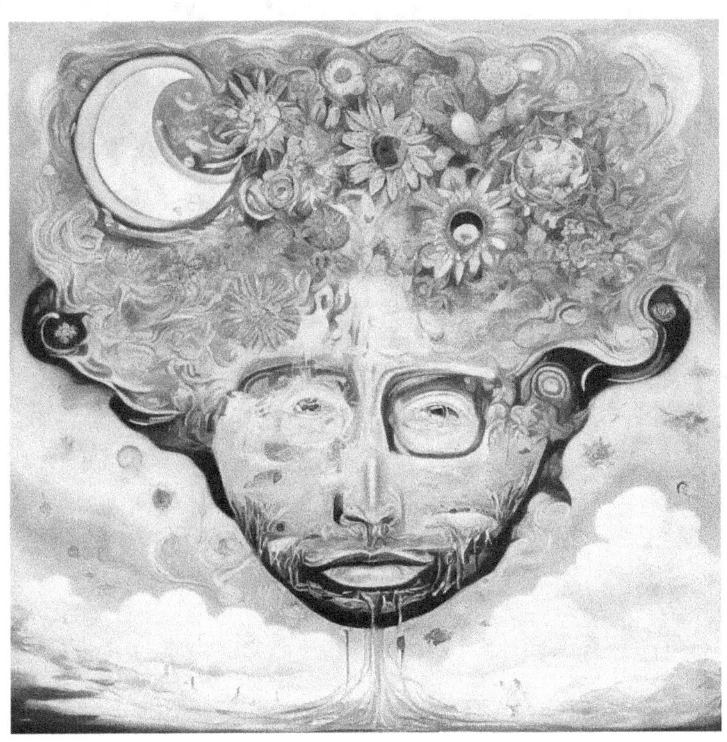

Acid Trip

Acid Trip - No not back to the 70's

Not to late – Go with FOLATE – vitamin B9: folic acid,
WARNING: synthetic form: dihydrofolate (DHF): causes a
disturbance in lipid and energy metabolism and disrupts normal -
GOOD FOLATE (natural) - 5-methyltetrahydrofolate metabolism
– Farmers spray synthetic folic acid on plants to help them
germinate but now there is an overuse everywhere and concerning.
 The concern: research has found associations between the folic acid
(synthetic) and increased cancer risk nothing more needed to say.
 NATURAL the way to GO - Folate is a vitamin B - folate binds to
folate receptors on our cells whereas the synthetic badboy hinders
and disrupts the natural process.
 Natural B9 FOLATE – Is present in green leafy vegetables, fruits,
and legumes in the diet – B9 helps the body make healthy new cells.
5-MTHF (5-methyltetrahydrofolate) IS the predominant
physiological form of folate found in blood and in umbilical cord
blood.
This is the B9 supplementation to utilize as it is the most absorbed
and methylated so no side effects!
 Check supplementation chapter on active B9.
 Why is this important? If trying to get to your perfect weight you
want to avoid another land Mine so eliminate something that causes
a fat disturbance. Aderailment of the energy of the cell the Badboy
folic Acid, so quit trippin.
Added note - Folate is important for the **synthesis and repair of
DNA**, other genetic material, and folate is necessary for cells to
divide. Go with FOLATE

Declaration: Put your Hand on your Heart and say:

"The Power to do anything stems from LOVE."

Acid Trip

CODE: TWENTY

You are A Sponge BOB square pants

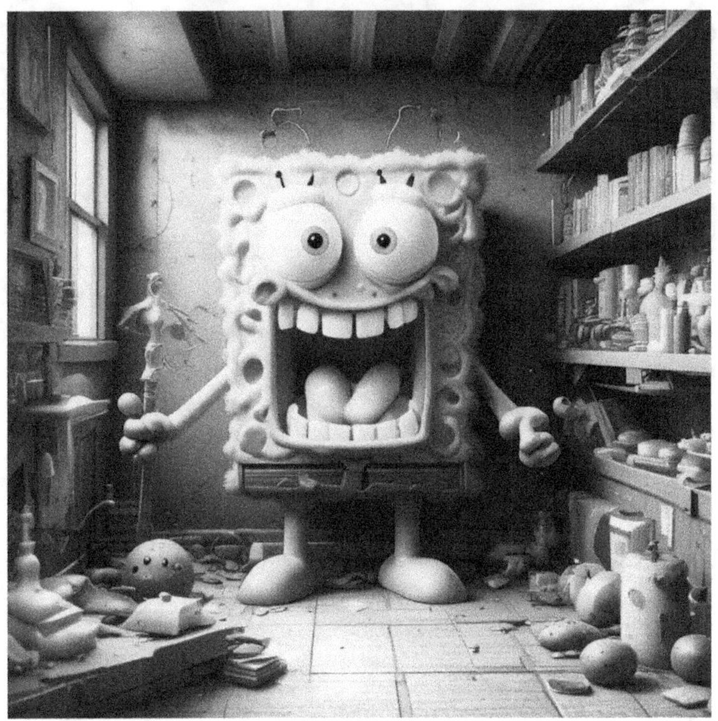

You are a Sponge BOB square pants

CRACKING THE FAT CODE

You are A Sponge BOB square pants

You Are What You Absorb and for 30 plus years I've been telling customers and clients "it's not what you eat it's what you absorb."

 If you're not breaking down your foods, they're not much use to you and sometimes you just need a little help.

"Yes With A Little Help From My friends" - Sgt. Pepper's Lonely Hearts Club Band, Beatles Album:
Yes more music in my head I can hear this amazing song as I write this.

This is really where EPIGENETICS come in to play.
 In the past customers would come into the store grab a product and give it a try, then days later coming back and and convey that the product just didn't work.
We would say ok and kindly give them a refund if they wished.
Now fast forward to This Day and I respond with much more clarity do to the understanding of the big picture of epigenetics.
My retort now is - It's more likely the product didn't work because your body and the fact it didn't absorb it, and or something else in your (epigenetic) environment has caused it not to work effectively or not at all and this is 97% of the issue.
Sure does make more sense now thankyou epigenetics, Dr. Lyons with Cell Well-Being, and Dr. Lipton.

 The bigger picture the "Epigenetic picture" that's numeral UNO #1 of what we should be focusing on saving you money and time in the long run.

You are a Sponge BOB square pants

The Help is from little **superhero enzymes** that can lend a helping hand PROTESE,LIPASE, and AMYLASE.

Enzymes help break down your foods.

Three main enzymes:

Protease breaking down proteins.

Lipase breaking down fats.

Amylase breaking down carbohydrates.

 This of course is all dependent on what kind of food you are eating, sometimes all it takes is just a quality digestive enzyme these little superheroes can help things along their way.
Important to note - Digestive enzymes also needed if normalizing candida overgrowth and for this they should be taken between the meals.

My story - I love cabbage rolls, but in the past, they didn't love me and I do enjoy them. Every time I had cabbage rolls or broccoli, cauliflower or Brussels sprouts I felt like I had a gas balloon or football in my stomach very uncomfortable, and if I passed Gas ,well who knows what would happen if the all the gas escaped at once, use your imagination or well maybe not..
 I rarely had these foods as much as I loved them knowing the health benefits they brought me, I just passed on them, instead of passing GAS with them.
Once I learned the importance of digestive enzymes, TADA Gas attack averted and no uncomfortable issues at all…

CRACKING THE FAT CODE

Now I just use a digestive enzyme when I eat the foods that may cause the possible disruptions in the digestive system.
They do help break down in the system and they don't cause any gut issues. They enhance your abilities not deter your body from normal function.

 I don't use digestive enzymes all the time but if I know I'm going out for a big banquet and know there will be lots of heavy food that I don't normally eat I bring digestive enzymes along with me. Truly amazing the difference when you utilize this and will help you along your way to your optimal weight as well nutrient absorption.

Another thing to share here when you are in that state of discomfort there is one product that stands out in the supplement world 100% natural called **Digest FORCE** – check it out in the Supplement Codes.

   Sometimes we need to repair gut issues, seems like everybody has IBS or some other digestive issue yeah, the nice thing about it is there's great options naturally to help repair the digestive system without harsh chemicals. my favorite being **Gut- FX** which helps heal the gut and intestinal lining. Checkout the supplement Codes for more info.

Declaration: Put your Hand on your Heart and say:

" I manifest My Life Naturally."

You are a Sponge BOB square pants

CODE: TWENTYONE

The KEY Masters

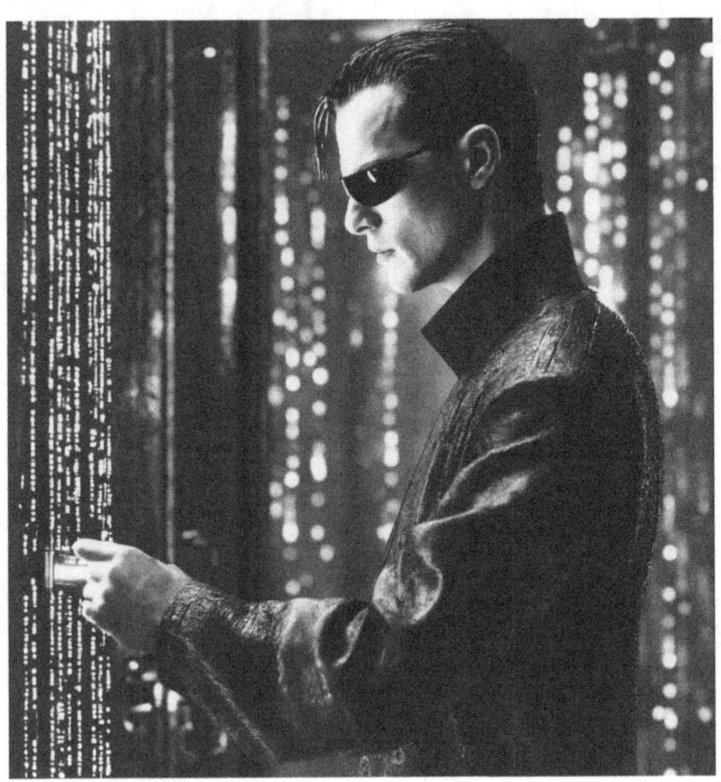

The KEY Masters

CRACKING THE FAT CODE

Key Masters

Thyroid: thyroid's function is to regulate the metabolism of the body. Like in the movie the Matrix they where looking for the Key Maker the Key Master who unlocked the door to the source. The Thyroid is very much THAT.
It's a master hormone and controls almost everything, iodine deficiency is one of the big reasons we become FAT. Within the thyroid, specialized cells convert iodine and the amino acid tyrosine into T3 and T4. There are no substitutions if you don't have enough iodine in your system, your thyroid absolutely cannot produce these hormones. Get enough Iodine and a great way for this is SeaSalt make sure a good sea Salt like REDMOND Real Fine Salt
Excess estrogen levels cause the liver to produce high levels of TBG thyroid binding globulin it binds the thyroid hormone and decreases the amount of thyroid hormone available to the body.

Ok Men take note, studies show in North America that Men at the ripe ol age of 75 have more estrogen than a woman of the same age. Are men more woman than a woman at that age? Yikes!

We are talking Xenoestrogens, fake estrogens – After entering the body they increase the total amount of estrogen resulting in a phenomenon called, estrogen dominance. Xenoestrogens are not biodegradable, so they are stored in our fat cells.

Buildup of xenoestrogens have been indicated in many conditions including: breast cancer, prostate and testicular cancer, obesity, infertility, endometriosis, early onset puberty, miscarriages, and diabetes.

Ultimately, the best way to support thyroid health is to live an overall healthy lifestyle. Drink plenty of water (not TAP water) this is one of the biggest culprits for estrogens!

Exercise regularly and reduce stress whenever possible. Iodine, selenium, iron, and zinc are all essential minerals for supporting thyroid health.

A way to get to the Source is using keys to unlock the power by a great Thyroid support product One being - Thyrodine - check in the supplement codes for more information.

Declaration: Put your Hand on your Heart and say:

" I LIVE a FEARLESS Lifestyle."

CODE: TWENTYTWO

Beige FAT is where its AT

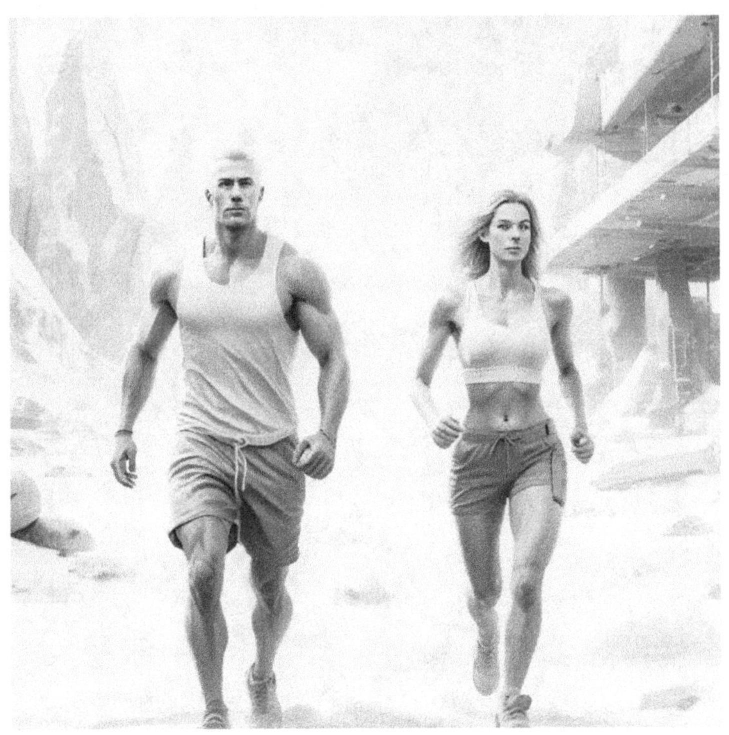

Beige FAT is where its AT

CRACKING THE FAT CODE

Beige FAT is where its AT

All FAT Not all bad or created Equal and the body Needs Fat every cell has a fat membrane with our Brains being approx. 60% FAT. Yes we are Fat Heads .
Guess what there, is more then just 1 type FAT
  Also, Fat tissue comes in an array of colours: white, brown, beige, and even pink.
The 2 main FATS being White and Brown
Let's start with Brown fat. It doesn't change with increased calorie intake, people that are overweight or obese carry less brown fat than their lean counterpart.
 So is brown better? Well brown FAT helps turn food into heat so I'd say YES.
Brown FAT breaks down blood glucose and FAT molecules to create HEAT revving up your metabolic engine ..so here WE go get your body working for itself!

Cold temperatures activate brown fat, which also helps to increase your metabolic state in the body. I am sure by now you have heard of the big jump towards, pun intended, "The Ice Cold Plunge"!
Mentor world Class Speaker, and motivator Tony Robbins does this everyday to get his Cells Revved Up!

The next Fat type is White the most abundant type and designed for fat storage this the pantry for storing calories, accumulating in the belly, thighs, and hips yikes I can almost hear the boos out there.
 but wait there's some Importance here, White FAT cells are needed and help produce around 50 types of hormones. They help process enzymes and Growth Factors (they act as communication molecules between cells including: leptin - primary role is to regulate energy balance).

Beige FAT is where its AT

 Moreover, White Fat helps our liver and muscles respond better to
insulin.
So here is the thing if there are excess White FAT cells the hormones
are disrupted and can cause a resistance (insulin resistance) and yep
chronic inflammation.
 It's all about balance.
The next type, the superstar – "You're the One That I Want" - I
know another song, sorry , not sorry I love music but fitting since its
from GREASE..lol.

 The one that we want more of because the metabolic change is
happening and more science discoveries are around this type
The new Brown is……..BEIGE
This FAT type is called BEIGE FAT this type of white fat converts
and performs like brown fat generating during cold temperature –
Oh ya the Ice thing again
 (this is where the whole cold showers or ice plunge aka Wim Hoff
the iceman, come into play to burn calories)
YES in addition to BEIGE FAT is used when we ..oh NO! Yep you
knew I was gunna say the "E" word again - EXERCISE .
Yes exercise so you just can't not exercise this is so key. Like the say
move it or lose it and in this case lose the ability for the FATS to
work in concert to bring all the FATS into harmony -Just like you
want your Body to be in – HARMONY!
When the body is cold, BROWN FAT is activated to use sugar, fat,
and amino acids from the blood to generate heat, Aton of research
has been done on this and more is coming out daily..

The Next Fat colour. Ok Gents skip through this paragraph
not for the guys just the ladies.

 PINK FAT another type of white fat that is converted to pink
during the pregnancy and lactation, producing and secreting breast
milk isn't the human body amazing!

Essential fat– Made up of brown, white, or beige fat and is vital for normal body function.
Found in muscles, organs, and the central nervous system most importantly the brain.
Essential fats regulate estrogen and other hormones, also helps with absorption of some vitamins and minerals.
Lastly then there was the dawn of EFA supplementation and the study of the importance of these Fats, We had the honor to have A leader in this subject Udo Erasmus on our radio show "Ask The Experts" and also a segment on the "wellnesswithkim" Radio Show!
 He wrote the the book "Fats That Heal Fats that Kill" an amazing resource Udo has been a promoter of EFA's and is world renowned as a matter of fact He was instrumental on the producing of the machines that extract the EFA's to be put in various products that many enjoy in their supplements around the world to this day.
A great product line for healthy EFA's in helping to regulate and help with many of the above activities is : at welnesswithkim.ca
Specifically one of my favorites checkout the supplement section.

 NOTE: Eating too many calories in the long-term can cause fat cells to increase in size and be stored in various areas throughout the body, which leads to that risk of chronic inflammation and the glitches in healthy metabolism

Declaration: Put your Hand on your Heart and say:

" No matter what I eat my Body can assimilate it."

Beige FAT is where its AT

CODE: TWENTYTHREE

The Sponge and the Chimney Sweep!

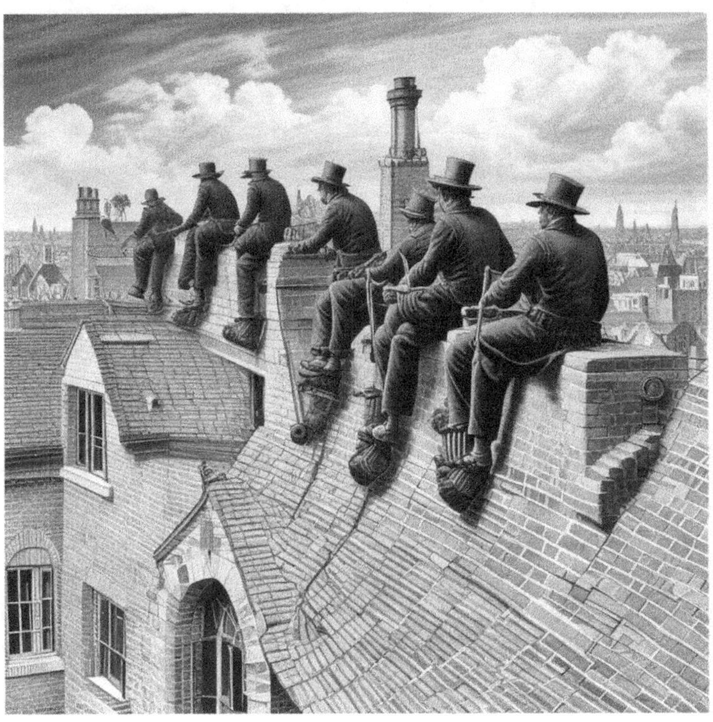

The Sponge and the Chimney Sweep

CRACKING THE FAT CODE

- The Sponge and the chimney sweep!

Dietary Fibre
Fibre is very important for the human body it helps keep our
digestive system healthy and it helps with reduction of constipation.
Those that partake in a high fibre diet can actually reduce the risk of
heart disease, stroke and bowel cancers.

The Sponge and the chimney sweep is a focus on the soluble and
insoluble fibre.

Soluble fibre dissolves and breaks down in water and when it breaks
down it forms like a gel and acts like a **sponge** absorbing the toxins to
help the body release them out of the gastrointestinal track.
Insoluble fibre many call roughage does not dissolve in water and it
does not breakdown in your digestive system it passes through the
GI track pretty much intact, it moves the bulk through the GI track
and actually balances the pH in the intestines this helps promote
regular bowel movements.
It's kind of like the broom or the chimney sweep and clears away
toxic waste as the soluble fibre travels through the digestive track.
 A key and great benefit to fibre being in the diet is the fact that one
gram of fibre release seven calories out of the body, bonus and
SUPER helpful!

The Sponge and the Chimney Sweep

Years ago in a radio station far, far away there was a disturbance in
the air waves
Our radio show, "WellnessWithKim!"
 We had Dr. Brenda Watson as a REGULAR yes pun intended,
every Tuesday we used to call it "poop Tuesdays."
Dr. Brenda was the head of a digestive care company a naturopathic
Dr. and colon therapist, look her up she has some great books
relating to the GI system. much of our knowledge and leading us to
do the research came through Dr. Brenda and her mentors including
Bernard Jensen the father of Iridology in North America.

 Some foods with the **sources of fibres**:
 I will start with my favorite,in which I have already spoken about
which are hemp hearts we get our hemp hearts from Rocky
Mountain Hemp out in Alberta Canada. Hemp hearts are both
soluble and insoluble, but this great superfood is amazing for protein
and good fats as well and should be a staple of everybody's diet.
 Some other **soluble fibres** include beets, apples , carrots, lentils, oat
bran, peas, peaches and oranges.
 Konjac root or Glucomannan a superb natural fibre sometimes
seeing it in the market place as a supplement called PGX this is a
remarkable product and again should be part of your daily
consumption.
 The **insoluble fibres** include
 Hemp hearts (both soluble/insoluble) steel cut oats, flaxseed,
cauliflower, potato skins, wheat bran and whole grain pasta to name
a few.
I must say all of the above should be of a quality source non-GMO
organic.
 You should have nothing but the best for your body mind and soul.

Declaration: Put your Hand on your Heart and say:

"Changes are Fun and Rewarding."

CODE: TWENTYFOUR

Beam Me up Scotty!

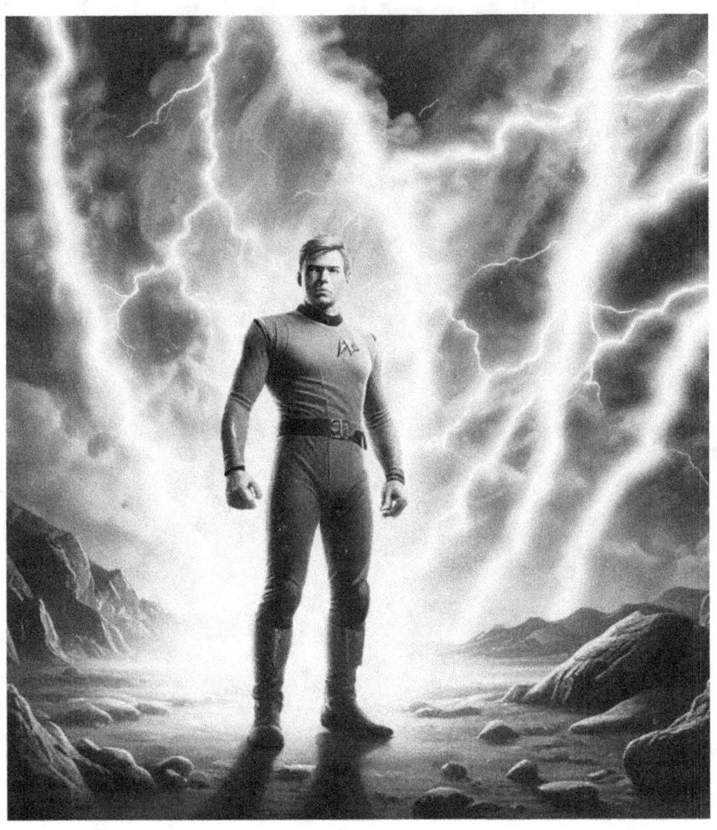

Beam Me up Scotty!

CRACKING THE FAT CODE

Beam Me up Scotty!

EMF's and EMR's, Electro Magnetic Fields(frequencies, forces) Invisible hazards?
Researchers have shown that 35% of people in developed countries suffer from chronic sensitivity to EMF waves. Because of these invisible hazards our body mechanisms slow and sometimes shut down causing many health issues including Cellular Fat gain.

I knew a little bit about these EMF hazards around 2001 but it wasn't until 2004 that I really got involved and dove deep into this issue that we're in now.
Back in 2004 I went to a conference in Toronto ON Canada and some EMF/EMR specialists/scientists from California came up and talked about these invisible hazards wow what an eye opener!

I gained a lot of knowledge and the one thing that stood out to me made a lot of sense. These gentlemen ascertained that you could be taking in all of the healthy foods, living a healthy life, eating organic, taking in different supplements in spite of this your vitality, health not increasing and optimizing.
Here's the AHA moment, they explained if your body is being bombarded 24/7 the body does not have time to relax and it is under constant stress, so the body doesn't know what's friend or foe.

Beam Me up Scotty!

The body puts up a shield and doesn't let all the nutrients in.
 The more substantial AHA to me was the fact that the body doesn't
let the TOXINS out, BIG AHA and BIG KEY!

Every living thing has a bio field some people call it an aura
and there are several frequencies around us some can harm some
heal us. I increased more knowledge on the Bio field and frequencies
when I became a vibroacoustic therapist some years ago.

Back to 2004 We were given a DVD from Australia it involved a
group of people that we're trying to stop a contractor from building
homes under power lines.
 In the Video they were holding up fluorescent tubes, these tubes
we're lighting up under the power lines as the people held them, they
looked like lightsabers from Star Wars. I've always been a healthy
critic and skeptic, so I needed to try this myself, with my wife and
our son we ventured forth to a local area where we knew a few large
homes sadly built near sizable power lines and we proceeded to do
the same test.
 We donned our Light Sabres (the fluorescent tubes) and sure
enough they lit up in our hands under the power lines, crazy town
wow it worked they glowed in our hands just like the folks in the
video from down under.

 We learned later in doing some research in the area that two of the
homes that were very close to the power lines had multiple families
that lived there, all of the families had cancer in the households,
more than so some food for thought there.

 I always tell people NOW to do your research and try out these
things, word of caution we felt sickly the next morning almost like
flu like symptoms so for this proceed with caution.

CRACKING THE FAT CODE

Soon after this I was given a book "Invisible Hazards In The Wireless Age" by Dr. George Carlo, In this ground breaking book he showed the effects of electromagnetic frequencies any electromagnetic radiation.

Doctor George Carlo was commissioned by the cell phone industry to prove cell phones were safe.
Now if we step back in time a little bit this was warranted due to a story (became a BIG story) that came out of Florida in the United States.
The husband went up against the cell phone industry, his wife died of brain cancer being a real estate agent she was always on a cell phone. When diagnosed and they showed the x-ray the tumor in her head look like the top of a cell phone with the antenna! No way...Way! This has been documented sure seems crazy but True.

After she passed He fought like heck, He got all the way to the Supreme Court of law and of course lost, he was up against a lot of deep pockets but what did happen is he got on Larry King live who had a lot of listeners.
The cell phone industry needed someone who knew about EMF's and EMR's to come to the rescue.
Stage left -Enter: Doctor George Carlo (NOW,a world recognized medical scientist, best-selling author and attorney. His career spans thirty-five years and more than 250 medical, scientific, and public policy publications in the areas of public safety, health care, consumer protection and human performance.

Beam Me up Scotty!

Before and At the time Dr. Carlo, being one of the brightest in the
science of the Wireless and Electro pollution conundrum, was asked
to show Cell-Phones were SAFE.
So after a year or so he came back and told the industry they
wouldn't like his answer and he told Them a resounding YES there
were enormous RISKS with children and major health issues with
Cellphones and the EMF's EMR's.

Well. The multi Nationals really didn't like his answer as you can
imagine and He was given his walking papers.
Later down the road Dr Carlo of course was made out to look like a
quack and his findings dismissed!
There was way too much power and money at stake doesn't take a
rocket scientist to figure this part out, follow the MONEY.

Doctor George Carlos rebuttal was a whistle blower book called
"CELLPHONES – "Invisible Hazards In The Wireless Age"
released Feb 12 2002.

So as this happened and after us doing our little experiment, I talked
to other people that knew about these stress induced issues caused by
the electromagnetic energy around us and over time WE found
Solutions to the issues.

A little EMF/EMR history, around 200 years ago circa 1900 there
was around 3000 EMF's and EMP's and our body could handle that
amount of EMF/EMR stress very natural no issues.
In today's age there is, are you ready for the Number....
Ready, set, son of a Gunshar, over 40 trillion. 40 TRILLION
EMF/EMRs!
Dancing around wave after wave hitting our Bodies Electric System
and stressing the body's cells 24/7.

CRACKING THE FAT CODE

The Ailments that arise because of these new age ailments are as follows:
chronic fatigue syndrome (CFS)chronic pain
tinnitus
depression
hormone dysfunction Alzheimer's disease
leukemia
Hard science linking all of these. Now with 5G upon us and I tell people don't do it!
Seems 5G will have a massive impact on the outer one to two inches of our bodies because of the shorter wavelengths and rapid absorption according to preliminary findings.
The 5G predictions are :

Blindness
hearing loss
skin cancers
male infertility
autoimmune conditions
thyroid issues

Whether this will happen or not, from my vantage point and with all of the Bio Hair scans I have provided thousands over the last seven years with clients, witnessing in the report the priorities of EMFS/EMR's, I advise for people to limit the time on these devices. Let these devices enhance your life don't let them own you, it's unfortunate devices ARE owning most people and harming them.

Beam Me up Scotty!

Parents PLEASE keep cell phones and tablets away from young children including baby monitors and cordless phones so many hazards that we don't realize. I am thankful that companies are out there to protect our loved ones.
One company I had the pleasure to doing a podcast with has done just this, finding solutions and bringing to the public products for helping keep people safe.
Backed by science and with impressive results.

 Being involved with the Wellness industry for over 35 years I am thankful and amazed of the people that I've met, crafting quality products and providing solutions to the public.

Most of the time the reason people get into the Wellness industry or produce a product is because of personal ill health issues with themselves their family or friends and they want to make a difference.
Change the outcome for someone else, find Solutions!
The owner Kim of the company mentioned above was one of these amazing people and he wanted to protect his family and others.
Kim back in the 90s was able to identify some crystalline properties while he was engaged in environmental cleanups in 1996 where he used a blend of materials to neutralize chemical and radioactive waste from landfills.
The paramedic substances worked, he then investigated to see if they would neutralize the EMFS for cell phones and other electronic equipment and voilà they 100% Do neutralize the harmful effects!
 He then soon after funded a research program at the quantum biology research laboratories.

CRACKING THE FAT CODE

I have seen amazing results when people utilize the devices that he designed and brought to the public.

I do something called the cell will being hair scans which takes 4 to 6 root bulbs of your hair preferably close to the brain stem and these Root Bulbs are placed on the S drive (based on Tesla coil technology) the hair follicles get digitized and sent to Hamburg Germany then sent back via a 36 page report with a 90 day program.

I then go over the report with my clients to start them with their Wellness journey. Over the last eight years when people have utilized these EMF harmonizers, we have seen significant change in the cell wellbeing epigenetic reports.

emfprotector.ca for protection from the 40 trillion EMF's and EMR's around Us everyday!
This should be one of your priorities not only for you for your loved ones.

If you want to getting to that perfect weight, then you have to address those invisible hazards that are constantly bombarding you every day. Getting devices devices that can harmonize those harmful hazards then the body can relax and do its job more efficiently.

For more research checkout Dr.Magda Havas from Trent University and for a video I had the pleasure to do an interview with Dr Havas go to https://www.youtube.com/watch?v=GM-fix7Mo10&t=6s

Declaration: Put your Hand on your Heart and say:

"TRUTH is the ONLY way."

Beam Me up Scotty!

CODE: TWENTYFIVE

Dive DEEP

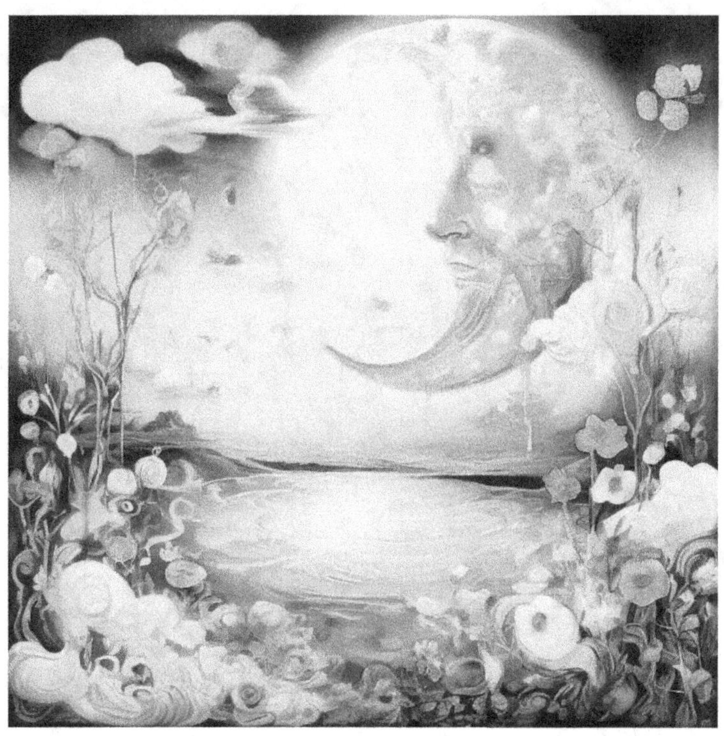

Dive DEEP !

CRACKING THE FAT CODE

Dive DEEP

Your Window to the The Universe

Nope not napping, caffeine, and that 'binge sleeping' on the weekend they are ineffective methods for recovery. The Only time our bodies Repair is SLEEP. Between the times of 10:00 pm and 2:00 am where the body goes through a spectacular process of physical repair. Between roughly 2:00 am and 6:00 am the body will go through an additional process of psychological repair. A disrupted sleep pattern will cause the Cortisol to elevate and negatively affect the regenerative process.

"poppies, poppies, poppies will put them to sleep, sleep now they will sleep"

-- The Wicked Witch.

So we need sleep to repair our bodies and not getting enough leads to weight gain.

Sleep Deep – In Delta WAVES "REM" sleep these are the most important brain waves to be swimming in. Your DELTA FORCE! The amount of sleep that you get is just as important as the proper diet and exercise studies have shown that those that don't get proper sleep stress more, burn less FAT and are more inflamed when they wake so quality sleep is crucial.

Dos and Don'ts to get that quality sleep is:

Turn all those electronics turn off disconnect the Wi-Fi or put a timer on it that it shuts down at a certain time.

Put your cell phone on airplane mode or have it in the next room any light in your room should be distinguished.

Blacking out the windows so it's pitch dark is best. Although I don't believe we should be working midnights we aren't bats still many people are on these shifts many black out their windows from the daylight to help trick the body.

Dive DEEP !

Since circadian rhythms are closely related to environmental cues
like light, they can affect how a person feels throughout the day.
Stop watching that TV and if you are then invest in some blue block
glasses for the evening. Science have shown that these do work and
help you get your circadian rhythm back to normal.
 Seven nights of too little sleep causes hundreds of genetic changes
and thus negative consequences and positive cellular FAT gained
which is what you don't want!
…Sleep is also the only time that We repair so it is essential to get
that REM sleep we all hear about.
 In 2014 I became a vibracoustic therapist and learned more about
those brain waves we hear about.

Every day we go through waves - The Beta waves the Alpha waves ,
Theta waves ,Delta waves and Gamma waves,
 Theta is that relaxed meditative state flowing into the dream state.
Alot of people do drumming ceremonies, If you've been around
when people are drumming you feel the thump thump thump in the
centre of your being. Many experts say drumming gets you into the
Theta state when you're relaxed.

Years ago historians remarked, that "Sitting bull"
the famous North American Lakota leader could get into the Theta
state and talk to animals, I find that kind of interesting.
Working with Dogs I know that your energy plays a big part with
how they react to you and respond to your commands.

Delta is the one we need to focus on for anti aging and weight loss it is the slowest brain frequency.

It's responsible for HGH secretion the human growth hormone which is directly related with body fat and muscle.

When in Delta your deepest phase of sleep is reached (REM) it's the doorway to your subconscious mind the key to collective subconsciousness. This is where we can change our negative thoughts to positive ones this is where the body heals and repairs itself.

Expert opinions:

Dr Amanda Mullin, Founder of Mindworx Psychology & Doctor of Clinical Psychology explains sleep isn't just necessary for the mind, in the body, the hormones that influence our weight get out of balance.

Dr. Merrill Milter a forensic examiner and expert in the physiology of sleep and fatigue states

"The fact is, when we look at well-rested people, they're operating at a different level than people trying to get by on 1 or 2 hours less nightly sleep."

"If you haven't slept, your ability to learn new things could drop by up to 40%."

From Dr. Mathew Walker from Neuroscience and Psychology at U.C. Berkeley and the founder of The Center For Sleep Science adds: "You can't pull an all-nighter and still learn effectively," Walker says.

Lack of sleep affects a part of the brain called the hippocampus, which is key for making new memories. Also "REM sleep helps take the sting out of emotional wounds so that you feel better about hurtful experiences the next day.

Dive DEEP !

From the Diabetes Journals:

 Sleeping in a cold room can help prevent weight gain, and even help you with weight loss goals. When your room is set to an optimal, cooler temperature, the melatonin your body produces will cause your body to store BEIGE FAT' which helps you burn calories instead of storing them.

 Helping repair and getting the Brain to homeostasis for the next Day is a Priority – Stay COOL!

A new tech that is just a patch with no chemicals or supplement it's
NERO TECH
 this Tactile device has benefited a lot of my clients to date and is taking the world by storm.
The Patch for deeper sleep is called REM from a company that started out of the GTA Toronto, Canada

Go to brainshift.ca for more info and give these tactile patches a try they have documented amazing results.

Declaration: Put your Hand on your Heart and say:

" I increase my Vibration of Love, Peace and Joy every Day."

CODE: TWENTYSIX

Order in the Court

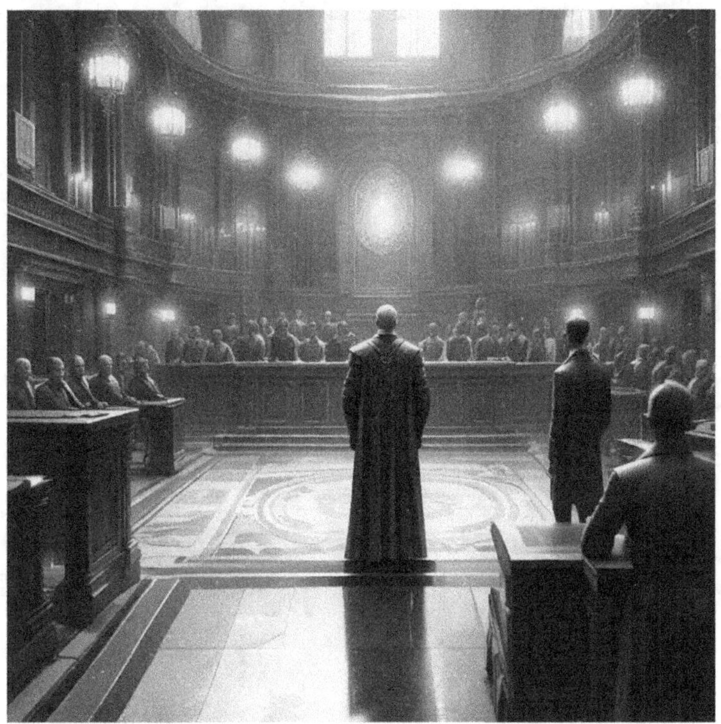

Order in the Court

CRACKING THE FAT CODE

Order in the Court – All rise !

All rise, well not so fast, we really don't want it to rise not for very
long anyways.
We are talking Cortisol:
Cortisol (from adrenal glands) - the stress hormone and one of the
chemical messengers.
 - Cortisol is both FAT storing and FAT releasing.
 Too much can cause havoc. The good part of cortisol meaning when
in balance with the body helps the body metabolize glucose and it
moderates blood pressure and blood sugar.
Cortisol when performing properly can also curb inflammation that
it also supports your immune system.
But under stress, chronic stress which causes high levels of cortisol
that's when everything gets out of wack!
The out-of-control cortisol contributes to weight gain especially
around the midsection and on the face.
High Cortisol can cause major fatigue, mood swings and produce
unwanted acne.

 There are many things you can do to relieve stress a lot the
suggestions discussed throughout this book will inevitably help with
adrenal fatigue and the elevated out of control cortisol in the body.

Declaration: Put your Hand on your Heart and say:

"My old Mental Scars are Gone."

Order in the Court

CODE: TWENTYSEVEN

Conquer Nature

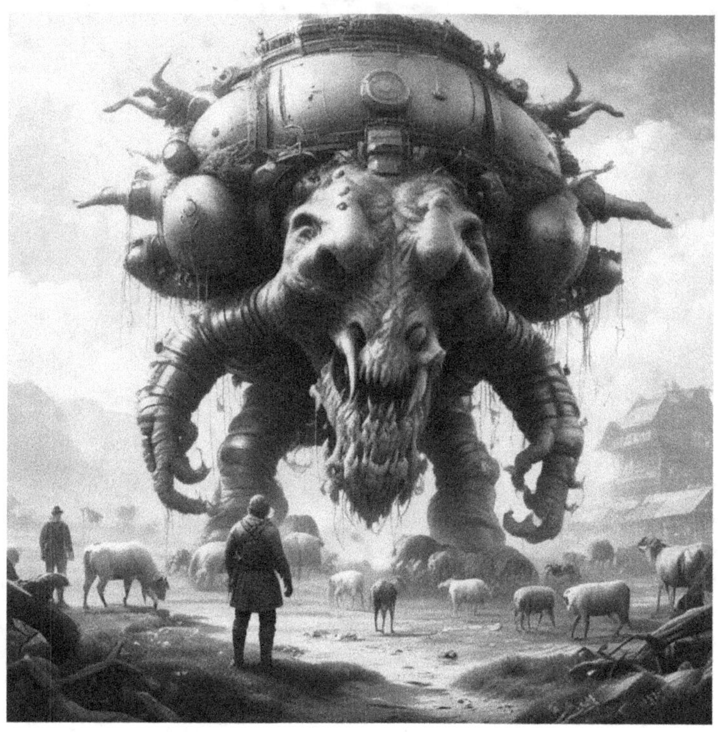

Conquer Nature

Conquer Nature

The Dictator - Big PHARMA

 Prescription drugs for everyday conditions cause you to gain a lot of excess fat many researchers agree that they a big contribution to the obesity epidemic

If you're taking a product that has 2 pages of side effects you really gotta take a hard look at it! For the most part people don't question, why not question it?
 At the end of the day your health and Wellness is up to YOU mot your DOCTOR.
 It's your choice nobody is gonna make you do anything you don't want to do right?
I don't know how many times I've heard over the years a client saying "my doctors going to put me on……..", "or my doctor said I have to!",
or someone's MD says "if I don't take this Med I won't be your my doctor."
Sounds kind of like a temper tantrum to me.
Last time I checked your doctor isn't God they should be there to assist you not demand what you do with your body.
Find a doctor that will work with you, your doctor is not going to be in the coffin with you and nor am I so choose wisely.

Everybody has an opinion, there are so many of them out there, but 1 thing BIG Pharma has never said is that their drugs cure anything they're only treating symptoms. ZERO CURES!

Conquer Nature

If you're taking 10 different pharmaceuticals how in the world can these pharmaceuticals all do their job correctly when they are fighting against each other for supremacy in your body. What a chemical nightmare!

Food for thought: Big Pharma - conventional Medicine will NOT make money if you don't go to them, correct?

This is absolutely correct it's unfortunate but true they are The SICK CARE industry not HEALTH CARE - They need sick people or they're out of business.

Why don't they like natural solutions? It's economically quite simple, If a $40 bottle of natural holistic pills can help with inflammation or alleviate a chronic issue within a few weeks or months how does that PAY $$$$ for a doctor, a nurse, technicians, specialists ,hospitals and equipment?

Back Surgery for instance costs $20,000 to $90,000 dollars depending on the procedure. Heart Surgery $11,000 to $35,000.

Drug company profits for 2022 were over 1 TRILLION Dollars! This is WHY they call the Natural/Holistic approach to healing quacks,charlatans, snake oil salespeople etc.

-They have to throw all the negatives at Natural/Holistic and keep people coming through their PHARMA DOORS

$$$$$$ money, money, money $$$$$

So, NO to NATURAL it can't support the MACHINE!

It can't so they have systems put in place to keep you in their SICK CARE system and therefore must say no to NATURAL,There is way too much MONEY to be made!

Do some deep research then do a gut check ,What Feels Right to YOU?

Then make an educate CHOICE your Choice no one else's.

I am not against doctors nurses or other medical people I'm against the system and I'm against what the PHARMA system has done to keep the GOOD HealthCare, caught in the Sick Care, people in the Big PHARMA Bubble.

CRACKING THE FAT CODE

I have a great admiration to the nurses and respect for first
responders they are the backbone of the conventional health industry
and most have big hearts and very compassionate people.
As far as Doctors, most went to school to be a doctor to help others
its unfortune in spite of that their hands are tide.
 They are overworked and can't spend any quality time with their
patients. You're allowed 10 minutes and one question, correct?
So Doctor's end up just handing over pills on a daily basis or pass
the buck - meaning send you to a specialist of some sort who in turn
either pass you off to another or they also hand you pills, creams and
or send you to surgery that for the most part isn't needed.

I have met many medical doctors that went against the grain and
tried to implement some natural remedies in their practice and had
their license taken. I have a lot of stories on this.
There is a new breed of doctor who is listening more and are
agreeing with their patients Nodding their head YES to their patients
taking supplements and trying natural remedies. These are few and
far between but I'm hopeful conventional meets natural and NEW
industries will be Born for ALL to have OPTIMAL Health for
LIFE!
Again, do your research there's a lot of information out there to
show the evils and other manipulation. Think about this, they say
Practice, a Doctor practices medicine. Key word **practice**, they are
practicing on you, that word says it all.

I hope in the future things are more cohesive and all of these
remedies and therapies can go hand in hand with the advances in the
medical science of today.

Declaration: Put your Hand on your Heart and say:

"All resistance is EGO trying to do things it's way."

Conquer Nature

CODE: TWENTYEIGHT

Let the Sunshine In

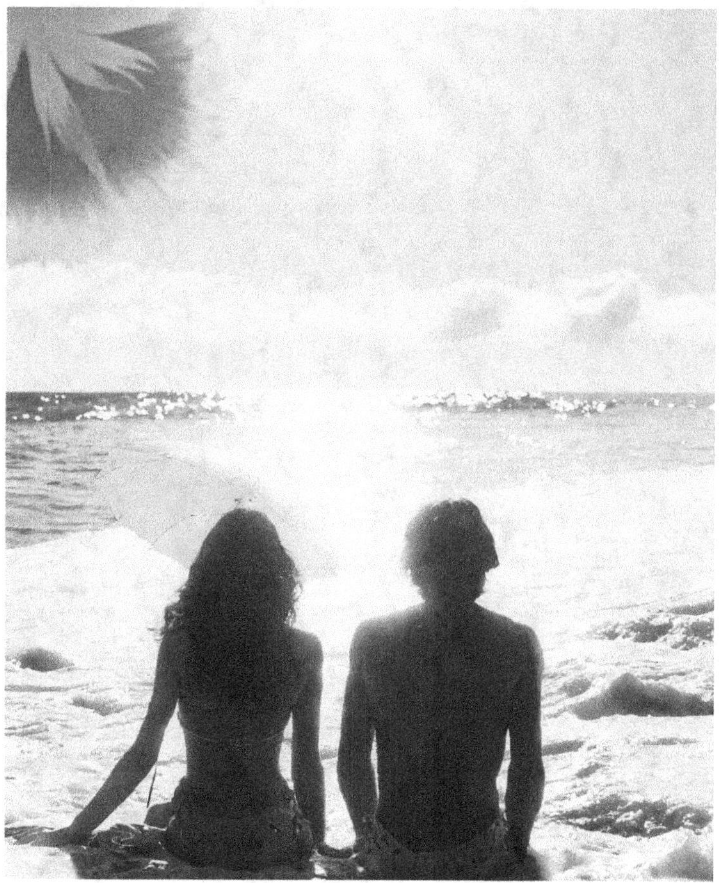

Let the Sun Shine In

CRACKING THE FAT CODE

Let the Sunshine In

Sunshine on my Shoulders make Me happy!
Not enough makes you sad and causes more issues than you think.
Lack of Vitamin D – in women, both total FAT and abdominal FAT
were associated with lower vitamin D levels, but that abdominal fat
had the greatest impact.

In men, however, lower vitamin D levels were significantly linked
with FAT in the liver and abdomen.

Packing on pounds in the winter?
Internal medicine reported that 77% of North Americans are
deficient.
From PUB Med evidence has shown that VDD (vitamin D
deficiency) is associated with extra skeletal conditions, such as
infection, cancer, diabetes mellitus (metabolic disease of type 1 and
2), cardiovascular disease, and autoimmune disease.

Just adding 5,000 IU's of a high quality Vitamin D which is
inexpensive will give you a much greater chance to achieve your
weight goals and make your much healthier.

Declaration: Put your Hand on your Heart and say:

"I am NOW fully Conscious of everything I Do."

Let the Sun Shine In

CODE: TWENTYNINE

Flow like Water

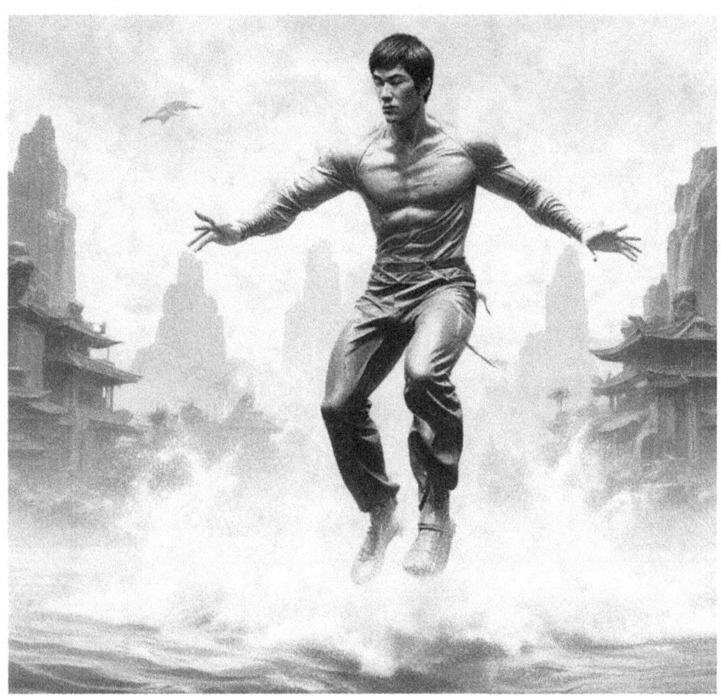

Flow like Water

CRACKING THE FAT CODE

"Flow like Water" - Bruce Lee

Poor circulation, helped by exercising and moving the blood through the 100,000 plus miles of our veins and blood vessels. Poor circulation can keep you from getting to your desired weight, regardless of your exercise or diet attempts.

Increasing the blood flow in brown FAT causes it to burn more calories in mice and may help treat obesity, a 2016 study in the Journal of Applied Physiology reported.

Sluggish like a wet sponge, slower circulation interferes with your body's FAT-burning processes.
So, circulation is key in getting that blood flowing there are many research studies with regards to copper and circulation.
Wearing copper like the items my friends at Newco naturals in Calgary Canada promote can help if need be.
There are different therapies like vibracoustic therapy and massage lymphatic drainage also to get the blood flowing. As well there are various quality supplements for Blood flow

Put your Health in YOUR HANDS!

Declaration: Put your Hand on your Heart and say:

"Expect a Miracle."

Flow like Water

CODE: THIRTY

Gut Check

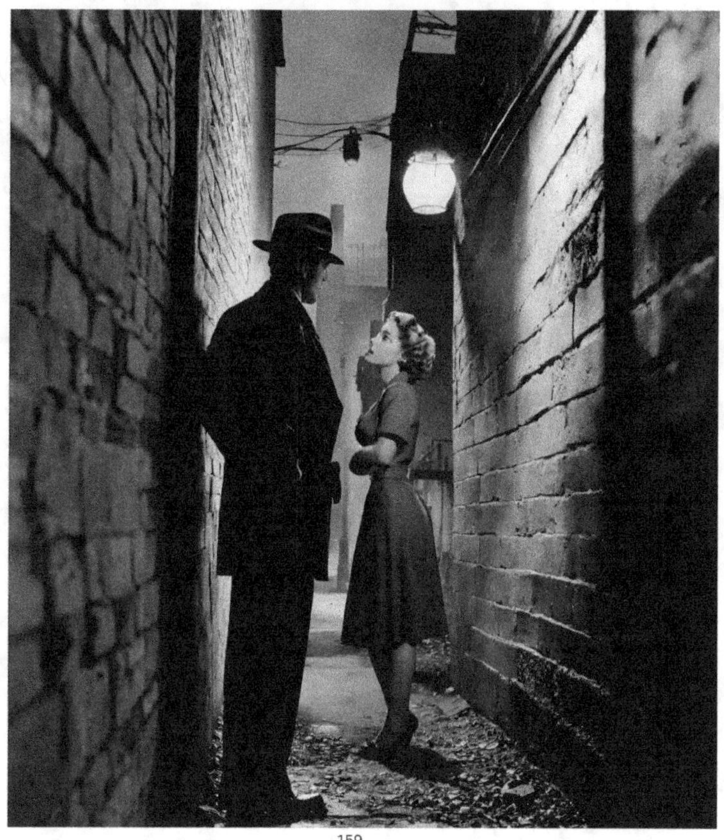

Gut Check

Gut Check

The Gut Brain connection - When we eat food, neurons in our guts send signals to our brain via a central "wire" called the vagus nerve.
 These signals send information to the brain about the nutritional value of the food and help regulate the brain's "reward" system in response to receiving the meal.
Different foods bring into play different influences on the gut/brain communication system.
 In A study, De Lartigue and team used cutting-edge technology to explore how sugars and fats can modulate this signaling pathway and thus influence our brain's reward center. They discovered two dedicated vagus nerve pathways: one for FATS and another for SUGARS.
These circuits, originating in the gut, relay information about what we have eaten to the brain, setting the stage for the cravings.
 The biggest take away I find is the following statementwhen we eat food, neurons in our guts send signals to our brain via a central "wire" called the vagus nerve.
 These signals send information to the brain about the nutritional value of the food and help regulate the brain's "reward" system in response to receiving said meal.

There is a lot of talk out in google world about MINDFUL Eating. It's about time!
More data on the Gut-Brain: Jan 18, 2024, Neuroscientists Discover the Gut-Brain Link Activated by Sugar and Fat

There are approximately 100 billion neurons in the human brain, your gut contains 500 million neurons, which are connected to your brain through nerves in your nervous system.
 The vagus nerve is one of the biggest nerves connecting your gut and brain. They found that distinct gut-brain pathways are recruited by fats and sugars, explaining why that dessert or trans FAT burger can be so irresistible."

 Ultimately this research provides insights on what controls "motivated" eating behavior, suggesting that a subconscious internal desire to consume a diet high in both fats and sugar has the potential to counteract dieting efforts. Neuroscientists Discover the Gut-Brain Link Activated by Sugar and Fat the vagus nerve signals information to the brain about the nutritional value of the food and help regulate the brain's "reward" system in response to receiving said meal. Different foods exert different influences on this communication system.
 In the study they use cutting edge technology to explore how sugars and fats can modulate the signaling pathway and thus influencing our brains reward centre.

Buy the Way - Neurons love Omega 3's and antioxidants, these protect your hippocampus from oxidative stress. Go for those Omega 3's instead of that Cake!

Declaration: Put your Hand on your Heart and say:

" I am now Free of all my negative thought Patterns."

CODE: THIRTYONE

Wonder Cells Activate

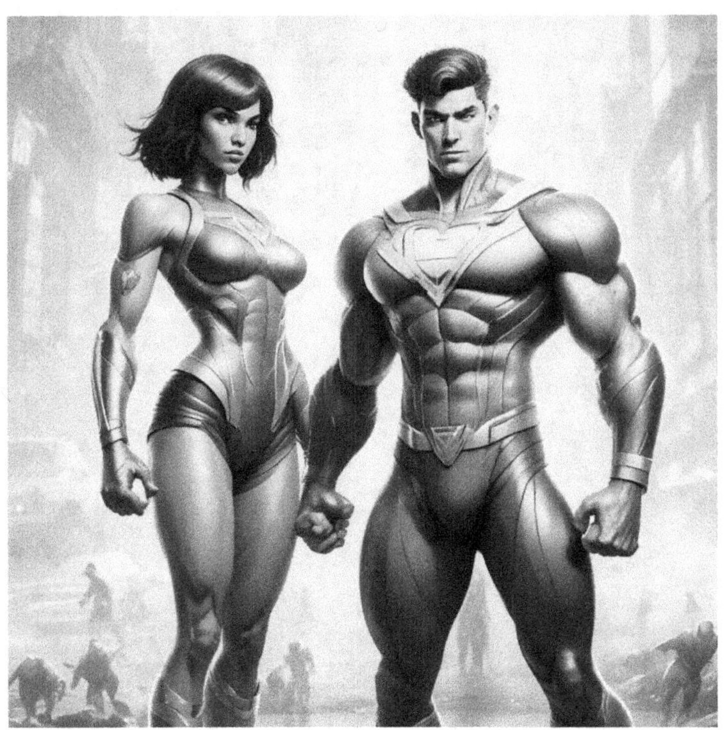

Wonder Cells Activate

Wonder Cells Activate - Power UP!

Supplement Activation
   Some still believe we don't need supplements well booo to them…
but hey 2 each their own. Abruptly I counter to those and say,
"I am a Believer ", I truly believe we do and they do a lot of good.
 I have been taking supplements since the early 80's and will continue
to take them until I expire in this life, they don't hurt you and at the
very least they give you some insurance and possibly up your game.
 They have done me well I've been able to do everything natural in
my life including bodybuilding, martial arts and other sports and
growing older gracefully. Along the way supplements helping me
repair my body without conventional means. I've went through three
doctors two have passed away and one is retired and I'm still going
strong at 59 years old.

 When I was 38 years old, I had 4 bulging disks and two herniated
discs, every four to six weeks my back would go out on me, I looked
physically strong and was but my back seemed to be my Achilles
heal. I had doctors fighting over me two said I needed surgery one
said I might be paralyzed if I got that surgery the other one said I
probably didn't need the surgery now but explained I had
degenerative disc disease and that I would probably need to have
back surgery down the road.
 Well, none of that happened hearing the possible paralysis scared
the hell out of me so I reacted with a great big NO!
During this same time in 2004 I was opening my first health food
store with my now wife Kim, a few months open this kind older lady
came in and introduced me to a coffee supplement, told Kim and I of
the benefits and what it had done for her.

Wonder Cells Activate

She explained the coffee was infused with beneficial medicinal
mushrooms (no not the magic ones) but nonetheless to me they were
magical, We agreed with her and said ok, purchased some, why not I
loved my Coffee but knew it was dehydrating to the cells.
 She assured Us this coffee was the only one that helped hydrate the
cells being an adaptogen and no the beverage doesn't taste like
mushrooms. Sorry I must always state this because everyone asks
cause nobody should mess with our morning COFFEE, right.

BAM ... in the short time my back ailment was over 80% better.
 My back is better now then it was over 20 years ago.
Every morning, I Enjoy my mushroom coffee with health Benefits!
check some out for your morning Healthy Coffee.
www.healthcoffee.ca

 I have so many other stories I could share that are very impressive
from clientele and customers and what they achieved through
supplementations. (Humm, another book perhaps?)

Athletes at elite levels and at the pro level take supplements of some
sort, that should give you a a clue and want you at the very least
consider them. All you have to do is do the research food generally
does not have the nutrient density that it once had.
 The soils are depleted, and a lot of the food is subpar, no we do not
live in the garden of Eden anymore. But what we need to do is to
make sure you're getting the supplementations that is beneficial for
you at the cellular level. There is so much in the market, Buyer
beware, do your research, go with Quality and NATURAL.

Ask Experts and those you Trust not a cheap big box chain store
bargain bin product. Products with fillers and byproducts on the
label that actually could do more harm then good.

CRACKING THE FAT CODE

Visit your local health food store and deal with someone you trust. I have some of my favorite supplements and brands I trust. We have had many customers and clients try these various Products and they All have had great results.

 I have researched countless products that were talked about on our Radio Shows from years past. I also worked for a nutraceutical company in the 90s and I saw the good the bad and the ugly and having health food stores, we needed to do the research for our customers and family so we've constantly done and continue to do the research.
For the most part I Now leave my supplement opinion out of it though and Wait.
I leave it to my S-Drive (Tesla Coil Technology) which provides the Cell Well Being Hair Scans.
I feel like Dr Bones on Star Trek with his tricorder …This is truly a gamechanger.
Being a practitioner for the last 7 plus year this Epigenetic Test takes my opinion and everyone else's opinion out of it, your cells tell Us what's going on at the cellular level!

 With the epigenetic reporting your cells tell YOU what is needed, from amino acids to vitamins and minerals to environmental issues including EMFS and even give YOU a 90-day plan of what to do. Side note NASA uses this technology for its astronauts to keep them on the right track.
 Its your GPS for Health and Wellness Optimization.
Last minute add on right before putting the book out
Cell Wellbeing *just launched two new Hair Scan Reports*
Anti Aging Report – Optimize Youthful Cells
and *Optimal Weight Report – Optimize Weight and Shape!*
Exciting - Can you say synchronicity.
I had no idea they were launching these New REPORTS and at the same time I was finishing my book! – Meant to BE!

Wonder Cells Activate

Supplements are just that, they supplement your daily food
requirements and can and will Optimize your cells.
Which one will and how much depend on your activity and how
healthy you are. If you have been ill and couldn't eat for a time well
you have some catching up to do.
 If you were in an accident and you were bedridden you most likely
will need to up your protein intake and other supplements which in
turn will get you back to homeostasis and back in business more
efficiently and quicker.
If you have an autoimmune disorder, we may have to start there.

 I always talk about and start with looking into the mitochondria at
the cellular level and the oxidative stress at the mitochondrial level –
Protandium a Nrf2 synergizer
– What is Nrf2? - a protein, naturally found within the body. Its job
is to help regulate the work of antioxidant proteins that can help
protect against oxidative damage.
 This oxidative damage can be triggered by injury and inflammation
and involves the production of free radicals.
The NRF2 pathway is part of a large system the body possess to
protect itself from damage. **PROTANDIUM** the only product of its
kind to date is incredible and scientifically proven to decrease your
oxidative stress and free radicals by 40% in 30 days.
More info on this incredible bio hacking product at
choices4wellness.com
There you will find this product and others including a great collagen
activator and skin cream with incredible before and after results.
One of my Favorite supplements – Enhancing and charging up the
ATP (Adenosine triphosphate) the molecule that carries energy
within cells – Creatine!

CRACKING THE FAT CODE

I could do a whole book on creatine, when working for a
nutraceutical company in the 1990s I probably sold the most creatine
to health food stores then anyone in southwestern Ontario, Canada
it was and still is my favorite sports supplement to date.
Creatine, is found naturally in muscle cells and to synthesize, it
requires three amino acids: methionine, glycine, and arginine with
the help of 2 enzymes, glycine.
It's Process:
 Amidinotransferase (AGAT) catalyzes helping the first step of
synthesis and Guanidinoacetate methyltransferase which controls the
second step of the process.

Once the process is complete your muscles produce the required
energy during exercise.
We generally have 1 gram to 2 grams of creatine if eating properly
daily and this truly isn't enough and more than not, we are in a
deficit with creatine.
Creatine speeds up muscle recovery helps with performance can
prevent muscle injuries. Other benefits studies show creatine helping
with diabetes osteoarthritis fibromyalgia and neurodegenerative
diseases.
Ok, ok, ok, you're probably asking does it help me get to my perfect
weight.
I retort with a thunderous YES.
 Creatine helps with building lean body muscle. Muscle is your
metabolic engine which helps your FAT cells burn efficiently which
in turn helps you get to your perfect weight, there's your sign.
Creatine monohydrate was the product with which all the science
was based and done in the early years with its the original and to me
still the one to stand by so don't get caught up in some of the 3rd or
4th generation this and that product with a lot of fillers and bogus
claims.

Stay Original - Here is a creatine product from one of the Companies I use to work for and a quality choice.
https://wellnesswithkim.ca/products/18905201?
_pos=2&_sid=ae0049c08&_ss=r
https://wellnesswithkim.ca/products/18905211_pos=1&_psq=creatin
e&_ss=e&_v=1.0

Another Product that gets your motor running and helps the brain also with inflammation helping at the mitochondrial level, called
RegenerLife Longevity
  I use this daily for cellular anti- aging and cognitive function since I have had several concussions over the years in sports and and doing dumb shit. I wanted something to help me repair and stay ahead of the game, age gracefully and know who I am and where I am at 80 years young.
  This combination is a targeted-nutrient mitochondrial support wellness optimization all-in-one packets formulated to support all aspects of healthy aging. I love it – makes life easy!
Each daily packet contains three different RegenerLife supplements – Mitochondrial Energy, NMNsurge, and Omega-3+D Ultra Strength – plus Quercetin LipoMicel Matrix for capillary health.
https://wellnesswithkim.ca/products/24228701?
_pos=1&_psq=regenrlife+long&_ss=e&_v=1.0

If there is Estrogen imbalance a great product developed from a close friend Is called Estrosense for women

https://wellnesswithkim.ca/products/28400451?
_pos=2&_psq=estrosense&_ss=e&_v=1.0

MaleEnergy for Men - balancing estrogen in turn helps the body utilize testorone more readily.
https://wellnesswithkim.ca/products/28410501?
_pos=1&_sid=b0fba7bb9&_ss=r
If a man, after taking the Male energy, needs some more power in his putter this is a great product to try, It could help you sink that Putt.
https://wellnesswithkim.ca/products/50800901?
_pos=2&_psq=testo&_ss=e&_v=1.0
Thyroid
Life Choice's Thyrodine -helps in the function of the thyroid gland it helps prevent iron deficiency and anemia. Helps to form red blood cells it helps to maintain immune function.
https://wellnesswithkim.ca/products/90507212?
_pos=4&_sid=06f911fc0&_ss=r
Sea Salt - https://wellnesswithkim.ca/products/90755110?
_pos=2&_psq=redmons+salt&_ss=e&_v=1.0
Digestive enzyme
https://wellnesswithkim.ca/products/16301501?
_pos=1&_psq=digest+best&_ss=e&_v=1.0
For Gas,bloating - Digest Force
https://wellnesswithkim.ca/products/28206101?
_pos=1&_sid=36de594ab&_ss=r
My favorite Cleanse from FLORA – 7 channels of Elimination
https://wellnesswithkim.ca/products/16703101?
_pos=2&_psq=flo&_ss=e&_v=1.0

Protein Shakes: The Best the number One on the market Today is again from one of my favorite formulators -It is the most absorbable and the closes to mothers Milk!
https://wellnesswithkim.ca/products/ultimate-high-alpha-protein-tropical-vanilla-750-gr?
_pos=1&_psq=ultimate+prote&_ss=e&_v=1.0

Wonder Cells Activate

My Second choice for a Protein Supplement

ALLMAX Isoflex - from the old Company I worked for in the 1990's with many flavors to choose!

https://wellnesswithkim.ca/products/18900111?
_pos=8&_sid=f1dc5fa50&_ss=r

Want A High-End Meal Replacement: Regenerlife
https://wellnesswithkim.ca/products/regenerlife-high-alpha-whey-
protein-meal-replacement-french-vanilla-885-grams?
_pos=3&_sid=f1dc5fa50&_ss=r

There are many More I haven't mentioned ,along the Wellness Road We may meet and I can possibly recommend some not mentioned above there are thousands.
.

Now remember I am NOT here to diagnose or treat anyone here.
 These are suggestions products that I have seen great results with customers and myself and there have never been any side effects whatsoever from any of the above products mentioned up to the date of this printing.

Declaration: Put your Hand on your Heart and say:

"I am WORTHY of ALL that I can Imagine."

CODE: THIRTYTWO

Less Is More

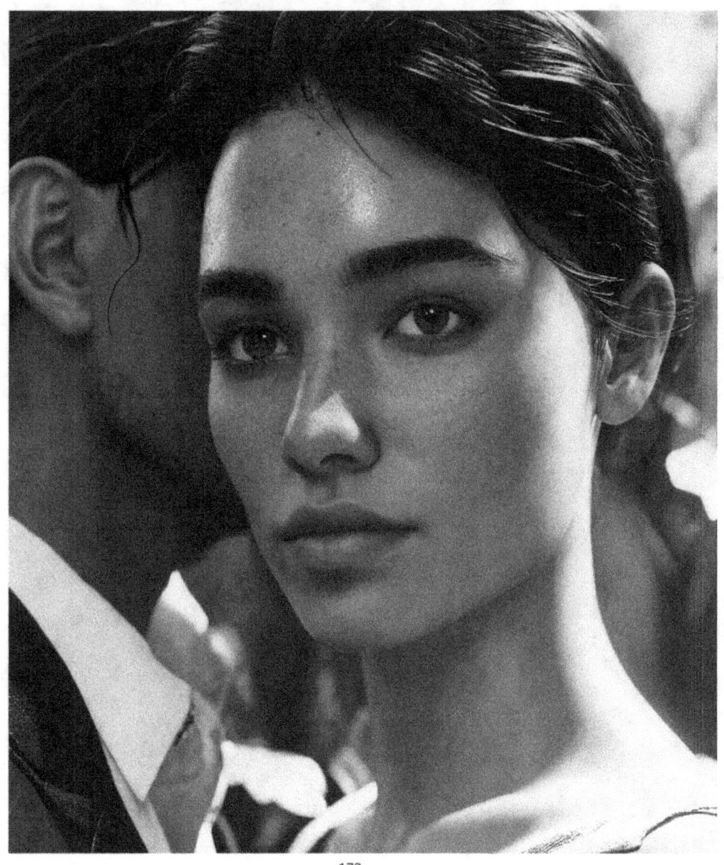

Less Is More

CRACKING THE FAT CODE

Less is More

Body care products,

This is a big one for ladies, but men should take heed as well! Less is more quite frankly there is not much need for a lot of the lotions and potions and certainly not antiperspirants sold on the open market.

First of all antiperspirants makes no sense as we need to perspire and the perfume's and smells that are chemically laden are hurting one of your channels of elimination part of the lymph system under your arms.

Body odor or B.O. is caused from an imbalance of pH remember everything from what you eat and drink, your medications, stress, hormones, and more can throw off your pH balance, causing a strong underarm odor.

There's a ton of toxic ingredients in most of the body care products in the market. In fact 5,000 tons of chemicals released in Californian homes documented in 2020

Look at the label and try to pronounce some of these chemical compounds. Good luck!

Check out the MSDS sheets on the compounds. A great resource for finding out about products and the ones you may be using is the Environmental Working Group

If you are putting a product on your skin your biggest organ make sure that is of a natural and non-toxic source.

You don't want your biggest organ the SKIN compromised, it being one of the seven channels of elimination for detoxifying.

Go Natural! Checkout: www.wellnesswithkim.ca for some great natural products

Declaration: Put your Hand on your Heart and say:

" I create my own challenges therefore I can create my own Solutions."

Less Is More

CODE: THIRTYTHREE

To Clean or Not to Clean?

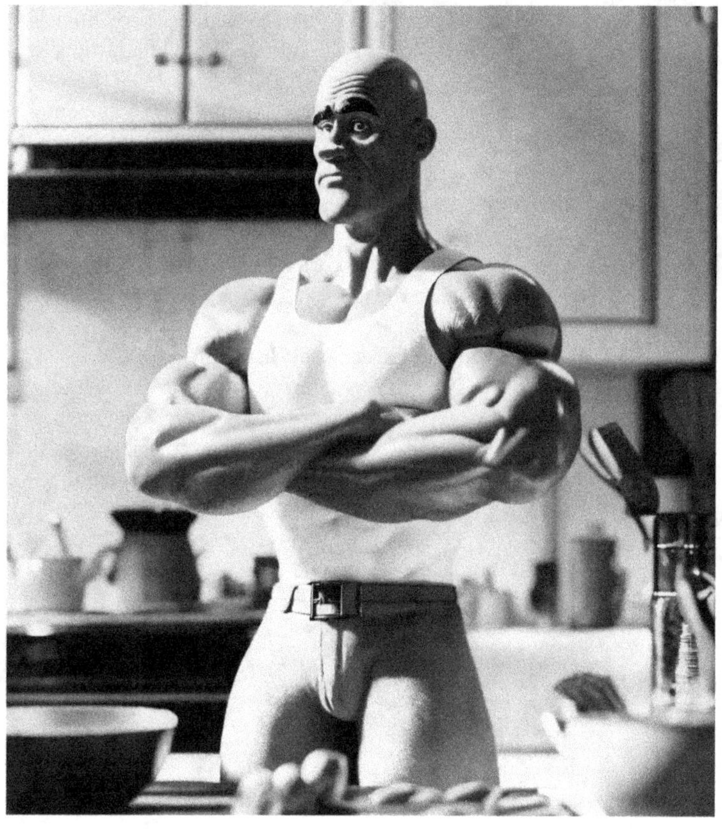

To Clean or Not to Clean?

To Clean or Not to Clean?

Cleaning products and cooking products in your home:
from laundry detergents and softeners, to kitchen, floor products to
Teflon or other aluminum cookware so many harmful to you, your
family, and the environment.
Not many know or even think to look at these items as a potential
threat we just go for the,"whats on sale" products, well that stopped
for me 20 years ago.
An eye opener is to watch the movie "Dark Waters" about Dupont
and forever chemicals. The environmental lawyer Robert Bilott,
spent more than twenty years litigating hazardous dumping of the
chemicals and blowing the lid off of PFOAS .

   Cleaning products can be expensive and very toxic to your family
and pets, from the synthetic Air fresheners to the essential oils in a
diffuser if of a low quality.
The last several years doing epigenetic bio hair scans I have seen
chemical hydrocarbons come up as a priority issue in many clients
and 1 of the reason for this is the overuse of essential oils.
I found this quite interesting, (NO I don't believe in coincidences),
that the whole FAD craze of essential oils was adopted around the
same time about eight years ago.

 My takeaway on this: use sparingly and use a very high-quality
product. Less is more!

Subsequently due to the Cell-Well Being hair scan reports we rarely use essential oils in a diffuser anymore.
We use Active Pure Technology (checkout the AIR CODE).
Surface cleaners should really be eliminated they cause skin issues to hormone disruption to cancer and other health problems.

Dr Doris RAPP(MD) environmental specialist, she made a mark and such a wealth of knowledge with many clinical videos on YouTube .
I am grateful and I had the pleasure of meeting her and listening to her lecture when she was in Toronto, Canada in 2004.
She put out very informative books and the One I tell Moms to read is:
"IS This Your Child" an eye opener for sure.
Adopt hydrogen peroxide, borax, baking soda and other natural cleaning sources.
Natural is the way. Cleaner, safer and cost way less money! You can eliminate all laundry soaps and softeners, dryer sheets and the toxic cleaners by installing an amazing product called
 Laundry Pro 2.0 with active pure technology and it will save you 500 plus dollars a year and can help the environment to boot. With an attachment on this device you can use the enhanced (hydrogen peroxide) water for cleaning everything in your home healthier and again saving you a lot of money.
https://aerusofwindsoron.com/laundry-pro/

Declaration: Put your Hand on your Heart and say:

" Imagination is more important than clean socks."

To Clean or Not to Clean?

CODE: THIRTYFOUR

Aerial Reconnaissance!

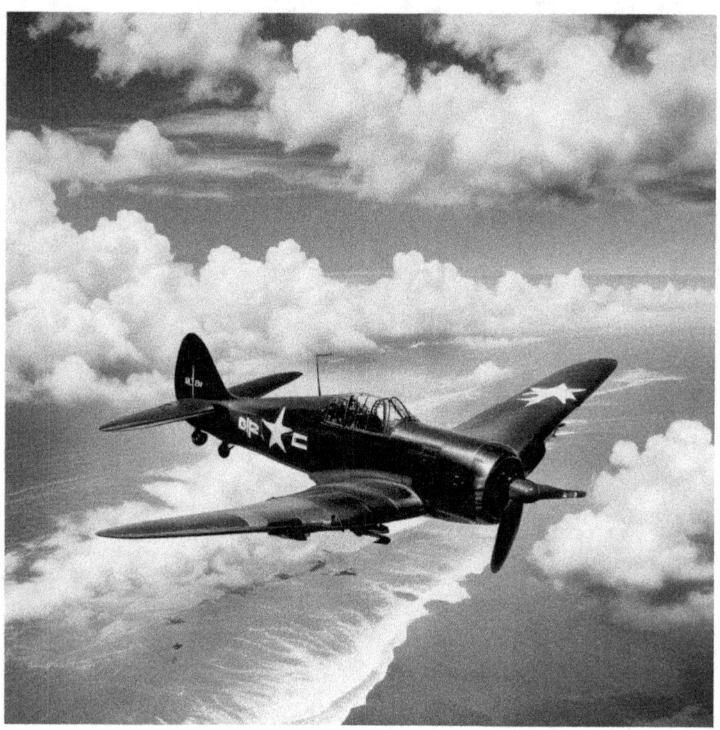

Aerial Reconnaissance

Aerial Reconnaissance

AIR - One of the Top if NOT top ELEMENTS for human Health and Wellness is also a major link in your Weight GOALS!
Science has established a strong link between air pollution and obesity. Breathing unhealthy air interferes with weight Loss.

Research reveals poor air quality is linked to obesity, heart and lung problems and metabolic dysfunction.
Exposure to airborne contaminants triggers a widespread release of inflammatory molecules called 'cytokines,'
The Cytokine Storms we keep hearing about which can increase fat storage, especially in the midsection.
Back to LEPTIN we talked about in another CODE.
 - Cytokines also increase inflammation in the area of the brain that regulates appetite and interacts with hunger hormones.
Resulting in a condition known as leptin resistance.
 Leptin is the hunger hormone that tells the brain you're full, so you stop eating.
 Inflammation makes the brain resistant to leptin's signals, which leads to overeating because you never feel full.
This a big Deal and needs to be addressed for FAT distribution and proper function.

A great resource for learning about Leptin is Dr. Robert Lustig, UCSF Division of Pediatric Endocrinology, Checkout his great video "Sugar: The Bitter Truth."
A study in 2020 – stated: Air pollution was linked to changes in the human gut microbiome which could fuel diabetes, obesity and inflammatory bowel diseases like colitis and Crohn's disease. We need Healthy AIR!

I love to cook and found this an important tidbit of info makes perfect sense. I have since changed how I do things in the kitchen. -Cooking can also generate unhealthy air pollutants from heating oil, fat and other food ingredients, especially at high temperatures. Also note that Self-cleaning ovens are shown causing weight gain. Open some windows if doing this function on your oven!
LOVE The Solution – High Quality AIR of course!
   We have been friends of https://aerusofwindsoron.com/ for seven years plus now and with Active Pure technology these various machines eliminate the pollutants, molds, pathogens everywhere in your HOME and Workplace.

– They are #1 in the WORLD. This year 2024 is their 100th Birthday....So happy Birthday AERUS!
 And I am thankful and grateful to talk about them, their products and technology.
Spreading the GOOD AIR news across the World...
This one FOR sure of the 1st steps to a Healthy HOME - Clean Healthy AIR!
Get a Filter or be the Filter your choice.

Declaration: Put your Hand on your Heart and say:

"I choose ONLY the BEST."

CODE:THIRTYFIVE

The Lawn Boy

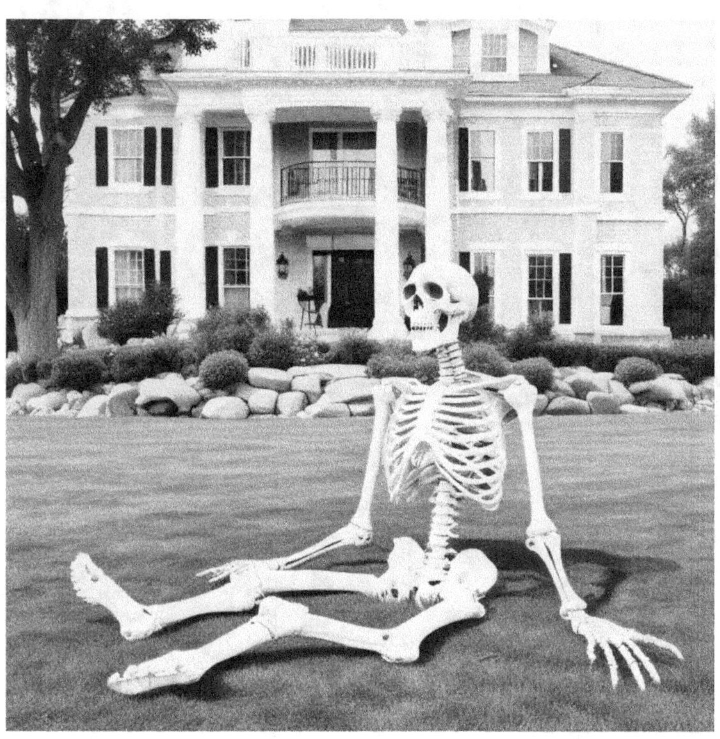

The Lawn Boy

CRACKING THE FAT CODE

The Lawn Boy

The history of the Lawn, check out the WEB when you do you will realize they are really just for show and not at all holistic or helpful. This CODE is not just for Us but for pets and nature to prosper. My Rant why LAWNS? We should change our thinking about Lawns,pesticides and your lawn. I know why its not being pushed hard for change ,Lawn and Garden Consumables worth USD 21.93 Billion by 2030!

100 million pounds of pesticides are used by homeowners in homes and gardens each year. Your grass may be greener than your neighbor's, but at what cost? A study of **9,282 people nationwide, found pesticides in 100% of the people after blood and urine tested.** The average person was carrying around 13 of 23 pesticides tested. Pesticides sprayed on lawns cause issues by mimicking human hormones such as estrogen, these endocrine disruptors are suspected of causing fertility problems, miscarriage, reduced male birth rates, brain abnormalities, miscarriage, behavior problems, cancer, and impaired immune function! Is this the Cost you will accept for your Green Lawn? This is not only a cause of estrogen dominance but is leaked into our water systems and causing major harm to the aquatic life and also your pets. The Pets are walking across these spaces, then they lick their paws. More and more animals are getting tumors and skin issues because of the pesticides in neighborhoods across North America. If you don't have cows, or your lawn is a golf course then why do you need a lawn anyways?

How about butterfly gardens, small ponds and plant herbs that help us, keep Us healthy and nature around us.

This is one way we help ourselves our family and the pollinators.

Declaration: Put your Hand on your Heart and say:

"Faith , sometimes , is doing the right thing no matter WHAT!"

The Lawn Boy

CODE: THIRTYSIX

Operation Minesweeper

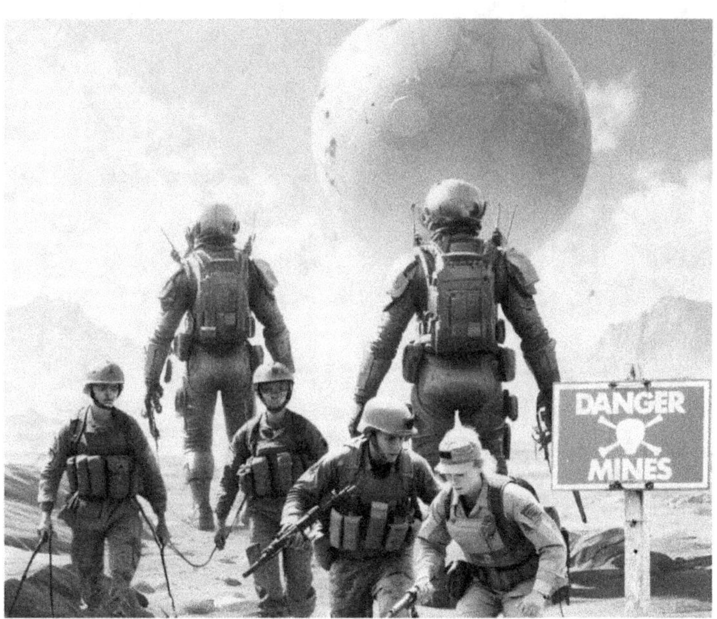

Operation Minesweeper

OPERATION MINESWEEPER

All in all it's the ENVIRONMENT you are Living In
The petry dish you put your body in daily.
 Change the environment and you finally get to your Perfect weight
not onlythat the Healthy vibrant body you want.
 "change your Petri dish change your LIFE!"
Wow ... A lot of Land Mines EH!
However for every land mine there are many solutions so these
CODES are kinda your personal minesweeper.
No need to be overwhelmed all of the Land MINES can be taken
care of as you maneuver through them.
 Some can be quickly taken care of where as others in time
 but all of them can be remedied.
Making use of all the CODES will get you to your optimal weight
and your Healthiest LIFE!
Your Brain/Mind Flow -
"The communication between our gut and brain happens below the
level of consciousness," since epigenetics dictates over 95% and your
genes approx. the 5% remember.......
YOUR subconscious mind (below the level of consciousness)
IS the FOCUS
- WHAT happens in your Inner world creates your outer world!
This makes sense why it takes such an effort to break through this
barrier and why 95% of weight loss diets Fail.
Well NOW You Know - HABIT- HABIT- HABIT
 Change your habitual environment utilizing All of the above
CODED information - Then.....YOU CRACKED THE CODE!
 "Fall in love with your body, its the beginning of a lifelong love
affair with magnificent, regenerative, optimal wellness."

One last thing – probably the most important aspect of living this life
is to ....**Be Grateful!**

Operation Minesweeper

CRACKING THE FAT CODE

Be grateful where you're at right NOW.
Be grateful what has happened in your life and what you've learned through your life to this point.
Be grateful for where you're going for the future is unknown…
I am so Grateful you read this BOOK!
 If you live a life of love peace joy and gratefulness you know where you're going…
Live your BEST LIFE God bless!
 In Optimal health and abundance,

Raimond Strazdins

This last declaration I dedicate to my boys, We said this together, very night before I tucked them In to bed when they were young.. Love you boys, where ever you are!

Declaration : Hand on your heart and say:

"I am happy healthy strong and grateful full of love and light"

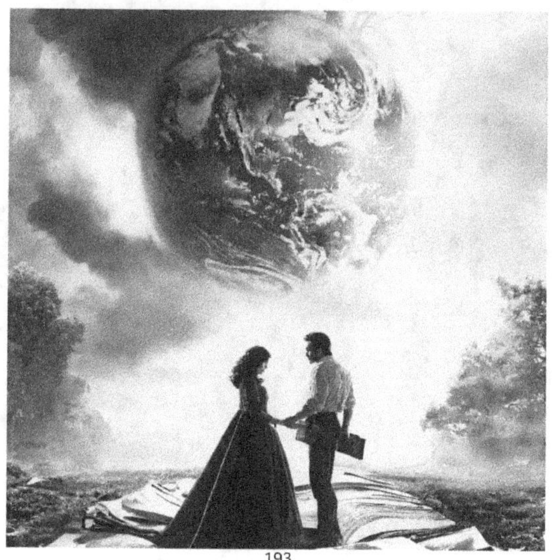

References

Sources:

#1 Source

Our many years of experts on OUR radio shows we were blessed to have them and gave me immeasurable tools to help Us help others – Thankyou ALL.

Other Sources:

www.nih.gov/news-events/nih-research-matters/how-brown-fat-improves-metabolism

ncbi.nlm.nih.gov/pmc/articles/PMC7739317

ncbi.nlm.nih.gov/pmc/articles/PMC9573946

ncbi.nlm.nih.gov/books/NBK551501

pubmed.ncbi.nlm.nih.gov/31939704

ncbi.nlm.nih.gov/books/NBK285545

ncbi.nlm.nih.gov/pmc/articles/PMC280570

Sources

https://www.ncbi.nlm.nih.gov/pmc/articles/PMC3262611/
https://www.nih.gov/news-events/nih-research-matters/gut-microbiomes-differ-between-obese-lean-people

https://www.medicalnewstoday.com/articles/321851#Vitamin-D-and-belly-fat-exposed Sutherland, L. N., Bomhof, M. R., Capozzi, L. C., Basaraba, S. A. U., and Wright, D. C. (2009). Exercise and adrenaline increase PGC-1{alpha} mRNA expression in rat adipose tissue. J. Physiol. 587, 1607–1617. doi: 10.1113/jphysiol.2008.165464 https://longevity.stanford.edu/lifestyle/lifestyle-pillars/lifestyle-medicine-sleep/

https://newsinhealth.nih.gov/sites/nihNIH/files/2013/April/NIHNiH Apr2013.pdf

https://newsinhealth.nih.gov/2013/04/sleep-it

https://www.mindworxpsychology.com.au/why-we-need-sleep-and-how-to-get-some/

https://diabetesjournals.org/diabetes/article/63/11/3686/34165/Temperature-Acclimated-Brown-Adipose-Tissue

https://www.ncbi.nlm.nih.gov/pmc/articles/PMC4390184/

https://pubmed.ncbi.nlm.nih.gov/38242133/

References

Sources

https://www.ncbi.nlm.nih.gov/pmc/articles/PMC7102907/

https://pubmed.ncbi.nlm.nih.gov/15242101/#:~:text=Aquaporins

https://pubmed.ncbi.nlm.nih.gov/21394604/
theconversation.com/brown-white-and-beige-understanding-your-bodys-different-fat-cells-could-help-with-weight-loss-138141

canada.humankinetics.com/blogs/excerpt/energy-systems

thorne.com/take-5-daily/article/benefits-of-alpha-lactalbumin-whey-protein

news.umich.edu/exercise can modify fat tissue-in ways that improve health

avivahealth/blogs/articles/cleansing-detoxification

The-History-of-Flor-Essence-Tea-a/256.htm

apathtonaturalhealth.com/blog/is-candida-making-you-fat

lpi.oregonstate.edu/mic/vitamins/folate

todaysdietitian.com/newarchives/111609p38.shtml

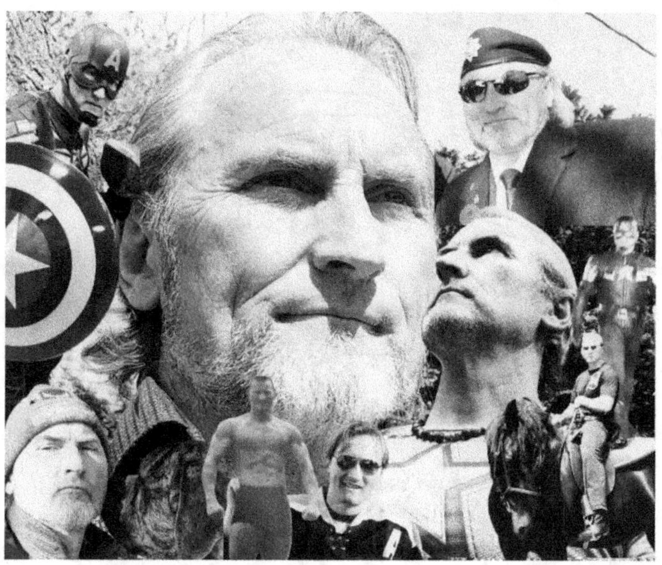

About the Author

Born: Raimond Strazdins, pen name
Adopted with given name Greg Foster
 Greg Foster, A nutritional researcher, holistic personal Trainer,
vibroacoustic Therapist and Cell-Well Being practitioner. Along the
way working for nutraceutical companies, co-hosting a radio show,
doing podcasts and owning health food stores and clinics. Writing
articles in magazines and newspapers over the years. Writing fiction
and non-fiction books and stories since the late 1980's
andNOWpublishing them many years later.
look for more books under
Raimond Strazdins